D1125608

CranioSacral

THERAPY

CranioSacral
THERAPY

WHAT IT IS

HOW IT WORKS

John E. Upledger, DO, OMM

with Richard Grossinger, Don Ash, and Don Cohen

North Atlantic Books
Berkeley, California

Copyright © 2008 by John E. Upledger et al. All rights reserved. No portion of this book, except for brief review, may be reproduced, stored in a retrieval system, or transmitted in any form or by any means—electronic, mechanical, photocopying, recording, or otherwise—without the written permission of the publisher. For information contact North Atlantic Books.

Published by   Cover design by Gia Giasullo
North Atlantic Books   Book design by Brad Greene
Berkeley, California   Printed in the United States of America

CranioSacral Therapy: What It Is, How It Works is sponsored and published by the Society for the Study of Native Arts and Sciences (dba North Atlantic Books), an educational nonprofit based in Berkeley, California, that collaborates with partners to develop cross-cultural perspectives, nurture holistic views of art, science, the humanities, and healing, and seed personal and global transformation by publishing work on the relationship of body, spirit, and nature.

North Atlantic Books' publications are available through most bookstores. For further information, visit our website at www.northatlanticbooks.com or call 800-733-3000.

Library of Congress Cataloging-in-Publication Data

Craniosacral therapy : what it is, how it works / John E. Upledger ... [et al.].
   p. ; cm.
   Most of the articles were previously published.
   Summary: "Presents writings by leading CranioSacral Therapy (CST) practitioners that explain the basic principles of this hands-on healing practice"—Provided by publisher.
   ISBN 978-1-55643-695-6
   1. Craniosacral therapy. I. Upledger, John E., 1932–
   [DNLM: 1. Manipulation, Osteopathic—methods—Collected Works. 2. Cerebrospinal Fluid—physiology—Collected Works. 3. Palpation—methods—Collected Works. 4. Sacrum—physiology—Collected Works. 5. Skull—physiology—Collected Works. WB 940 C8905 2008]
   RZ399.C73C69 2008
   615.8'2—dc22   2007050803

7 8 9 10 VERSA 20 19 18
Printed on recycled paper

North Atlantic Books is committed to the protection of our environment. We partner with FSC-certified printers using soy-based inks and print on recycled paper whenever possible.

Contents

Introduction

Throughout the course of human history, great discoveries have often been met with resistance before they have been accepted. Today we take for granted that the world is round. Yet to fifteenth-century citizens it was clearly flat, and anyone who sailed beyond its limits would vanish off the edge of the earth.

Now, as I look back over my own history of working in concert with the human body, I find myself at the summit of a body of work that collectively represents a tipping point in the acceptance of CranioSacral Therapy as a practical approach to the facilitation of good health. What was once considered unusual, even unorthodox, is gaining new converts every day.

As you'll see in the book you hold in your hands, there is good reason for that. From the scientific to the personal, these narratives bring to mind not only the great mystery of the human body, but ultimately the common sense behind its design.

Why should it surprise us that we can tap into the body's own inner wisdom to facilitate a positive response through the use of our hands and an innate desire to help? In my mind, this is health as it was meant to be—a natural collaboration between two human beings on a multitude of different levels, all simply allowing the body to do what it was born to do best.

I am honored to be with you at this point in history as we look toward a future in which we can learn new ways of supporting each other. It is time.

—John E. Upledger, DO, OMM

CranioSacral Therapy

JOHN E. UPLEDGER, DO, OMM

CranioSacral Therapy (CST) is a gentle, hands-on method of whole-body evaluation and treatment that may have a positive impact on nearly every system of the body. Whether used alone or with more traditional healthcare methods, it has proven clinically effective in facilitating the body's ability to self-heal. CST often produces extraordinary results.

CST helps normalize the environment of the craniosacral system, a core physiological body system only recently scientifically defined. The craniosacral system extends from the skull, face, and mouth down to the sacrum and coccyx. It consists of a compartment formed by the dura mater membrane, the cerebrospinal fluid contained within, the systems that regulate the fluid flow, the bones that attach to the membranes, and the joints and sutures that interconnect these bones.

Because the craniosacral system contains the brain, spinal cord, and all related structures, any restrictions or imbalances in the system may directly affect any or all aspects of central nervous system performance. Fortunately, these problems can be detected and corrected by a skilled therapist using simple methods of palpation.

By using about 5 gm of pressure, or roughly the weight of a nickel, the CST practitioner evaluates the system by testing for ease of motion and the rhythm of cerebrospinal fluid pulsing within the membranes. Specific treatment techniques are then used to release restrictions in

---

Reprinted with permission from Eric Leskowitz, ed., *Complementary and Alternative Medicine in Rehabilitation* (New York: Churchill Livingstone, 2003), 3–13.

sutures, fasciae, membranes, and any other tissues that may influence the craniosacral system. The result is an improved internal environment that frees the central nervous system to return to its optimal levels of health and performance.

The Scientific Foundation of CranioSacral Therapy

In its most basic sense the craniosacral system functions as a semi-closed hydraulic system that bathes the brain and spinal cord and their component cells in cerebrospinal fluid pumped rhythmically at a rate of 6 to 12 cycles per minute. To accommodate these pressure changes, the bones of the cranium and sacrum must remain somewhat mobile throughout life. The joints and their sutures do not fully ossify as was once believed. William Sutherland, DO, introduced this premise in the 1930s.

In the mid-1970s, Michigan State University (MSU) asked me to uncover a scientific basis for Dr. Sutherland's belief. From 1975 through 1983, I was Professor of Biomechanics at MSU's College of Osteopathic Medicine, where I led a team of anatomists, physiologists, biophysicists, and bioengineers to test and document the influence of the craniosacral system on the body. Together we conducted research—much of it published—that formed the basis for the modality I went on to develop and name CranioSacral Therapy, or CST.

We discovered that corresponding changes occur in dura mater membrane tensions as cerebrospinal fluid volume and pressure rise and fall within the craniosacral system. These changes in turn induce accommodative movements in the bones that attach to the dura mater compartment. When the natural mobility of the dura mater or any of its attached bones is impaired, the function of the craniosacral system and the central nervous system enclosed may be impaired as well.

Research Supports the Existence and Significance of the Craniosacral System

Studying bone specimens from live surgical patients ages 7 through 57 years, the MSU team was able to demonstrate definitive potential for movement between the cranial sutures.[1-5] Several other studies then laid the foundation for developing a model to explain the mechanism of the craniosacral system.

One important factor contributing to the MSU research was the discovery of what appeared to be fascia hanging from the free border of the falx cerebri on some of the cranium dissections that were performed on both embalmed and unembalmed cadavers. Under the microscope these tissues appeared to be nerve tracts running out of the falx cerebri with brain tissue attached to their free end.

Further research indicated they were components of a nerve impulse/message delivery system between these identified intrasutural nerve receptors and the walls of the ventricles of the brain in which the choroid plexuses were located. This research provided the basis for what our team named the Pressurestat Model, which explains the function of the craniosacral system as a semi-closed hydraulic system (Figure 1-1). Our findings supported those published in *Anatomica Humanica*[6] by Italian Professor Guiseppi Sperino, who noted that cranial sutures fuse before death only under pathological circumstances.

As a springboard toward the clinical application of therapy on the craniosacral system, an interrater reliability study was devised. Twenty-five nursery-school children were examined by two of four examiners on each of 19 parameters. The percentage of agreement varied from 72% to 92%, depending on the examiners and the allowed variance of either 0% or 0.5%.[7]

Subsequently, this same 19-parameter evaluation protocol was used to examine 203 additional school children. A technician recorded the

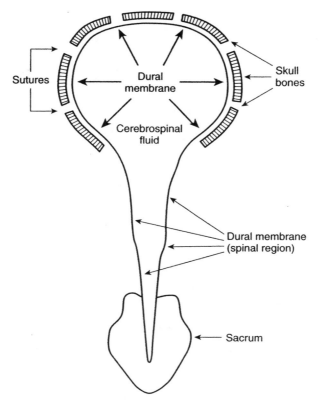

Figure 1-1 Semi-closed hydraulic system of the cerebrospinal fluid and dural membrane. (From Upledger, JE: *CranioSacral Therapy II: Beyond the Dura,* Seattle, 1987, Eastland Press.)

orally reported data for a statistician, who collected information from each child's school file and historical data from parent interviews. This information was compared with the craniosacral system examination findings.

The results of these studies showed that the standardized, quantifiable craniosacral system motion examination represents a practical approach to the study of relationships between craniosacral system dysfunctions and a variety of health, behavior, and performance problems.[8] Other researchers have done similar studies related to psychiatric disorders[9] and symptomatology in newborns.[1]

Craniosacral Therapy Encourages the Body to Self-Correct

CST is based on the idea that each patient's body contains the necessary information to uncover the underlying cause of any health problem. The therapist communicates with the body to obtain this information and helps facilitate the patient's own self-healing processes.

Thus the usual sequence of events carried out in conventional medicine is reversed in a CST session. Rather than taking a verbal patient history, the therapist begins through palpation, that is, touch. If the therapist is familiar with the patient's history before the session, he or she may find only what is expected rather than sensing the subtle clues offered by the patient's body, energies, and psyche. For that reason, patients are generally asked to write their medical histories and bring them to the clinic for their files. The therapist can then review the history later when he or she feels safe from the issue of suggestibility.

Although avoiding initial history taking is controversial, CST has been practiced this way successfully by tens of thousands of therapists since these concepts were first taught at MSU in 1976.

CST also diverges from conventional medicine in its approach to symptoms. Rather than trying to simply relieve symptoms, CST practitioners work to find and resolve the primary dysfunction underlying the presenting symptom complex. For instance, rather than seeing strabismus as a diagnosed condition to be corrected by surgery, the therapist searches for a cause within the intracranial membrane system and the motor control system of the eyes. In this case the cause is often found to be an abnormal tension pattern in the tentorium cerebelli.

Quite often these tension patterns are referred from the occiput or from the low back and/or the pelvis.

The CST "diagnosis" would be intracranial membranous strain of the tentorium cerebelli due to occipital and/or low back and pelvic dysfunctions resulting in secondary motor dysfunction of the eyes. Clearly in such a case the therapist would focus on the sacrum, pelvis, occiput, and then the tentorium cerebelli. Correct evaluation and treatment would be signified by a "spontaneous correction" of the strabismus.

A similar approach is used for almost any presenting problem, from TMJ disorders to recurrent bronchitis and spastic colitis. The nature of the presenting problem is usually of secondary importance unless immediate amelioration is critical, or if the patient does not understand CST. If this is the case, the therapist may attend to immediate complaints while patient understanding is developing.

How CranioSacral Therapy Differs from Cranial Osteopathy

CST is often compared with cranial osteopathy, which was developed by Dr. William Sutherland, the "father of cranial osteopathy." Although Dr. Sutherland's discoveries regarding the flexibility of skull sutures led to the early research behind CST and while both approaches affect the cranium, sacrum, and coccyx, similarities end at this point.

Today, as in the beginning, cranial osteopathy remains focused on the sutures of the skull. However, CST, as developed at MSU, focuses on the dura mater membrane system as the primary cause of dysfunction. The bones of the skull are involved only as they serve as "handles" for the practitioner to use to access and affect the membrane system that attaches to those bones.

Another major difference between the two approaches is in the quality of touch. CST practitioners generally evaluate and often correct imbalances in the system by using a light touch that has been scientifically measured between 5 and 10 gm, which is approximately the weight of a nickel resting in the palm of the hand. CST involves no invasive or directive forces but uses a gentle quality that often belies the effectiveness of the therapy. Most patients say they feel nothing more than subtle sensations during a typical session. In general, the manipulations used in cranial osteopathy are often heavier and more directive.[10]

Performing the Craniosacral Evaluation

During an initial CST evaluation, the therapist senses subtle motions while looking for any restrictions impeding free motion of the craniosacral system and various body regions, tissues, and organs, as well as the body's energies (Figures 1-2 to 1-4). The whole body responds to the rhythmical activity of the craniosacral system, which is evaluated for amplitude, quality, rate, and symmetry/asymmetry of response. Similar evaluations are conducted on the vascular and respiratory systems. The bodily responses, or lack thereof, to these systemic activities are significant factors in the search for the primary dysfunction.

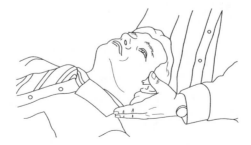

Figure 1-2 Palpating craniosacral rhythm at the head. (From Upledger, JE: *CranioSacral Therapy II: Beyond the Dura,* Seattle, 1987, Eastland Press.)

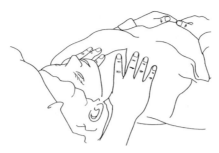

Figure I-3 Palpating craniosacral rhythm at the thorax. (From Upledger, JE: *CranioSacral Therapy II: Beyond the Dura,* Seattle, 1987, Eastland Press.)

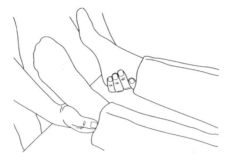

Figure I-4 Palpating craniosacral rhythm at the feet. (From Upledger, JE: *CranioSacral Therapy II: Beyond the Dura,* Seattle, 1987, Eastland Press.)

Another integral part of the initial CST evaluation involves the myofascial system. Fascia runs like a continuous web of tissue throughout the body and remains somewhat mobile under normal circumstances. Gentle traction applied on the fascia in arbitrary directions from various positions helps localize restricted areas. These areas of restricted mobility are then interpreted to be sites of either current problems or residue from previous lesions or problems.

Active lesions/problems are differentiated from inactive residual effects by a technique known as "arcing," which I developed with biophysicist Zvi Karni at MSU. By using mechano-electrical monitoring, we discovered that energies both within and off the body are palpable to the skilled therapist.[11] Arcing requires the therapist to sense the energetic waves of interference produced by the active lesion/problem; these waves tend to be superimposed over the normal subtle physiological motions of the body, organs, tissues, and energies. Practitioners then trace these waves to their source by manually sensing the arcs that they form.[12–14]

The source of the waves is considered to be the core site of the underlying problem or lesion, which may actually be quite distant from the location of the patient's symptoms. Usually the active lesion/problem disrupts gross physiological activities, as well as more subtle energy functions and patterns, such as acupuncture meridians.

As sites of dysfunction and disruption are discovered, the therapist may attempt to restore mobility to the involved tissues and energy fields. More often than not these attempts will be partially if not completely successful. In either case the result is often the appearance of a deeper problem or lesion for which the dysfunction just treated has served as an adaptation. The therapist then follows these clues layer by layer until the primary problem is disclosed. This may occur during the first evaluation or it may require more than one visit to bring the deepest underlying problems to the surface. In CST, it is necessary to clear the entire body of any mobility restrictions to achieve the highest level of craniosacral system function.

Most of this evaluation is carried out before the complete evaluation of the craniosacral system itself. Skilled therapists are encouraged to move in and out of the various body systems and regions, including the craniosacral system, as their judgment and intuition suggest. Peripheral body problems often refer into the spinal cord via their nerve root connections. The effect of these referrals on related spinal cord segments includes an effect on the dura mater, which is key to the function of the craniosacral system.

Correcting the Facilitated Segment

CST includes the concept that the dura mater membrane within the vertebral canal (dural tube) has the freedom to glide up and down within that canal for a range of 0.5 to 2 cm. The slackness and directionality of the dural sleeves allow this movement as they depart the dural tube and attach to the intertransverse foramina of the spinal column.

When nerve roots refer increased levels of impulse activity into the spinal cord from their peripheral domains, a facilitated condition of the related spinal cord segment occurs. A condition of hyperactivity in that facilitated spinal cord segment sends out impulses to the related dural tube and dural sleeves. The result is a tightening and loss of mobility of the dural tube related to the involved segment(s).

Clinical observation suggests CST is effective in releasing dural tube restrictions to normalize the activity of facilitated spinal cord segments. To locate these areas of restricted mobility, the evaluator tests the mobility of the dural tube and releases restrictions as they are found using gentle traction techniques. These releases are mandatory; if a peripheral restriction is released but the dural tube restriction and facilitated spinal cord segment are not, the peripheral problem usually reoccurs.

Once the peripheral body and the dural tube have been treated for restrictions, the therapist can focus on the cranium and sacrum. During this time the therapist also helps correct both primary and secondary dysfunctions of the skull bones, facial bones, hard palate, and sacrococcygeal complex. All related sutures and joints are very gently mobilized through the use of the bones as handles on the dural membranes inside the skull and spinal canal.

After mobilizing bony restrictions, the therapist then focuses on correcting abnormal dural membrane restrictions, irregularities in cerebrospinal fluid activities, and dysfunctional energy patterns and fluctuations related to the craniosacral system. At this stage the patient often moves from a phase of having obstacles removed to one of self-healing with the therapist simply facilitating the process. In essence the patient moves out of the realm of "fighting disease" into one of enhancing health. This self-healing is why CST is such an excellent preventive medicine modality—it mobilizes natural defenses rather than focusing on the etiological agents of disease.

A CASE STUDY

Vertigo in an Olympic Diver

Mary Ellen Clark was a world-class platform diver who had won several major competitions, including a bronze medal in the 1992 Olympic games in Barcelona, Spain. Not one to rest on her accomplishments, she had set her sights on making the 1996 Olympic diving team and bringing home another medal. She was in the best physical shape of her career. In spite of her age (she turned 33 in 1996), experts gave her excellent odds at accomplishing her goal.

Suddenly, Mary Ellen began experiencing vertigo, a condition that had ended the careers of several other divers she knew. Vertigo is a devastating condition for anyone and particularly for a platform diver. Each time Mary Ellen stood at the edge of the diving platform she felt off balance. Once she hit the water, she would become confused and disoriented, occasionally causing her to mistakenly swim to the bottom of the pool.

Mary Ellen saw many doctors and specialists and tried both traditional and unconventional treatment methods to find relief. Yet there seemed to be no solution to her problem. She was unable to train for 9 months because of the devastating effects of the vertigo, and she had all but given up her dream of remaining on the Olympic team.

In September 1995, Mary Ellen came to see me at The Upledger Institute Healthplex Clinical Services in Palm Beach Gardens, Florida. I started our first session by conducting a whole-body evaluation using my hands to test the mobility of the tissues and areas of restriction throughout her body. I quickly found several significant "energy cysts," or concentrated areas of foreign, disruptive, or obstructive energies, that likely resulted from traumatic blows to her body. Mary Ellen often did 50 dives a day from the 10-meter platform, and she hit the water at speeds of about 35 miles per hour. I used simple CST techniques to release her energy cysts manually without difficulty.

In the second session the CST evaluation pointed to Mary Ellen's left knee. She confirmed she had seriously wrenched it during a trampoline accident while practicing a new dive. At the time she paid little attention to the injury; she was accomplished at denying any presence of pain. As the evaluation continued, however, it became clear that the knee injury had caused a chain of compensation through her pelvis and lower back. Her spine had twisted to support her, which in turn caused her head to be improperly positioned on her neck.

As I helped Mary Ellen correct these problems, she began to improve. I continued to see her for at least one session each week for a straightforward combination of CST, knee and spine manipulation, pelvic rebalancing, and myofascial release. Within 30 days of her first treatment, Mary Ellen resumed her physical conditioning. Within 90 days she experienced a complete correction of the problem and was able to return to a full training schedule.

At the Olympic games in Atlanta, in July 1996, Mary Ellen Clark captured another bronze medal.[15,16]

A CASE STUDY

Intracranial Hemorrhage in a Newborn

Onar Bargior was born prematurely in Moscow, Russia, on February 7, 1991. He suffered severe cerebral circulation impairment, intracranial hemorrhage, and encephalopathy. He was diagnosed with infantile cerebral paralysis, spastic diplegia, and hypertension-hydrocephalic syndrome. Any stimulation produced muscle spasms that made his legs rigid and scissored, causing hyperextension of his truck and neck. His arms became rigid with clenched fists crossed in front of his body. Having almost no hip flexion, it was difficult for him to assume a sitting position.

In March 1992, Onar was registered as an invalid who could neither stand nor sit without direct assistance. His mother, Maiga, had tried to find help for her only son, yet medical treatment in Russia was limited and sporadic. Onar spent much of his life merely lying on a bed. Then a nonprofit medical relief agency in Waterville, Ohio, the International Services of Hope (ISOH), offered Onar and Maiga hope. ISOH specializes in bringing Third World children to the United States for donated medical treatment not available in their own countries. The organization has had remarkable success in securing life-saving and life-enhancing surgical and medical care for physically impaired or compromised children.

The agency arranged to fly Onar and his mother to New York for treatment at the Division of Pediatric Neurosurgery of New York University's Medical Center. Their clinical team evaluated Onar in October 1994. However, the doctors determined he was not an appropriate candidate for surgery and the subsequent rehabilitative care because of his extreme spasticity and psychomotor delays. The birth trauma and accompanying cerebral palsy had left his body too rigid to crawl or walk and had severely restricted the use of his right hand.

Onar's mother's hopes were shattered. Acutely aware of what this treatment meant to Onar, ISOH began to explore the availability of other medical care. In their investigations a representative consulted with a New York physician who had heard of an innovative program of care available through The Upledger Institute. ISOH contacted the Institute with the plea that the Institute was their "last resort." The alternative was to return Onar and his mother to Moscow without assistance.

The Upledger Institute accepted Onar into a 2-week intensive therapy program beginning March 13, 1995. This specialized treatment program is built around the use of CST complemented by physical therapy, Visceral Manipulation, acupuncture, massage therapy, play therapy, family counseling, and education. Onar's therapists consisted of a multidisciplinary team of physical therapists, occupational therapists, massage therapists, osteopathic physicians, and psychologists.

During Onar's first session, one of his therapists found severe restrictions in his dural membrane system—the falx cerebri, falx cerebelli, and tentorium cerebelli membranes inside the skull and the dural tube inside the spinal canal. She also found a compression of the sphenobasilar synchondrosis with a right sheer, ethmoid/frontal restriction with bilateral maxillary impaction and restrictions in the right temporoparietal suture, as well as the coronal suture. There were fascial restrictions in the cervical area relating to the hyoid bone, the sternocleidomastoid, and the suboccipital triangle muscles. The thoracic inlet and entire rib cage were restricted and rigid. There were also respiratory diaphragm restrictions with a visceral component into the stomach, and pelvic diaphragm restrictions with compression at the L5-S1 vertebral juncture. Treatment was applied to all of these areas.

On the second day of treatment, Maiga reported that Onar had slept soundly, which was an unexpected and pleasant surprise, since he normally woke three or four times a night. On awakening in the morning, he asked when he would be returning to the clinic. Throughout the program, Onar continued to show tremendous daily improvement, including an increased appetite, decreased spasticity, awakening without crying each morning, and increased range of movement of all joints.

Originally, the staff in Moscow and New York described Onar's psychomotor delays as so pronounced as to indicate mental retardation. Consequently, we were expecting a child slow to respond, both interpersonally and intellectually. What we found was quite the contrary. He impressed us from the beginning with his ability to communicate—initially through smiles, laughter, and emotional engagement. As he became more comfortable he began reacting in his native language, which was peppered with growing numbers of English words and phrases.

Coming into the program, Onar preferred to move by logrolling across the floor. The day he struggled to push himself up on his knees was another great milestone. He also began reaching for toys, and he developed the skills needed to play with stickers, little cars, and trucks.

The intensity of these programs and the systemic nature of the therapy they provide usually result in physiological gains continuing for several months after the program has ended. Because CST removes the restrictions that prohibit the body's natural inclination toward health, the body experiences a period of reorganization. Encouraged by such remarkable gains in Onar after just one treatment program, our staff decided to provide a second 2-week intensive treatment program after a 2-week period of rest.

The second treatment program began on April 10, 1995. To the delight of all involved, Onar demonstrated continued gains of physiological movement and decreased spasticity. On the second day of the program, when asked, "How are you today, Onar?" he answered in English: "I feel soft." On the fourth day of the program he was able to place his feet flat on the floor. By the end of the program he was crawling on all fours.

One of our physical therapists noted that, after the second 2-week session, Onar was using his right hand to reach and grasp objects with relative ease and accuracy. With minimal to moderate assistance, he was able to get into sitting, kneeling, and high-kneeling positions. He had not been able to perform any of these developmental gross motor movements before coming to the United States. Overall, his contracted musculature or spasticity had greatly relaxed.

When Onar first came to the clinic, his entire cranial system was extremely restricted and compromised. By the end of his second intensive-treatment program his cranial system was moving with greater amplitude and symmetry. This indicated that Onar's system was operating more efficiently and fluidly without many restrictions in and around his central nervous system. In time Onar was able to sit for longer periods, crawl with reciprocal movement, crawl in high-kneeling position with moderate assistance, and use his right hand without verbal prompting. He also began speaking more clearly and displaying a clarity of emotion and projection of love—traits most healthy children display.

By the time Onar completed his treatment programs he had also finished the necessary testing and inoculations to begin attending school. Maiga had worried that Onar might not be intelligent enough to get along in the world. But school testing showed that Onar has a fine mind. With opportunities for education, there is no telling what this child will do. He has already contributed in a profound way to the lives of his therapists and friends.[17,18]

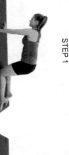

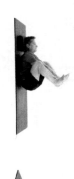

Movement
Slowly round your back up toward the ceiling, then let it sag down to the floor while looking up, and repeat.

Tip
Make sure to use your entire back for the motion and keep your movements slow and controlled.

Pigeon Pose
SETS: 3 | HOLD: 30 | DAILY: 1 | WEEKLY: 7

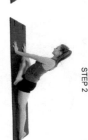

STEP 1

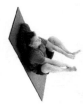

STEP 2

Setup
Begin on all fours.

Movement
Bring one knee up towards your arms and rest the outside of that leg on the ground, with your other leg straight behind you. Bring your trunk forward, with your arms straight on the ground, until you feel a stretch.

Tip
Make sure to perform this exercise slowly, and keep your back straight.

Supine Pelvic Floor Stretch
SETS: 2 | HOLD: 60 | DAILY: 1 | WEEKLY: 7

STEP 1

STEP 2

Setup
Begin lying on your back with your legs bent and feet resting on the ground.

Movement
Lift your legs off the ground with your knees bent and let them fall outward, relaxing your pelvic floor muscles.

Tip
Make sure to continue breathing evenly. This should be a gentle stretch.

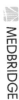
Disclaimer: This program provides exercises related to your condition that you can perform at home. As there is a risk of injury with any activity, use caution when performing exercises. If you experience any pain or discomfort, discontinue the exercises and contact your health care provider.

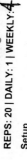

Quadruped Full Range Thoracic Rotation with Reach

REPS: 20 | DAILY: 1 | WEEKLY: 4

Setup

Begin on all fours.

Movement

Lift one arm out to your side, then to the ceiling, rotating your trunk at the same time. Next, reach that arm all the way under your body, through your opposite arm and leg, rotating your trunk in the opposite direction. Repeat these movements.

Tip

Make sure to keep your movements smooth and controlled. Follow your arm with your head as you move.

STEP 1   STEP 2

Supine Bridge

REPS: 20 | DAILY: 1 | WEEKLY: 3

Setup

Begin lying on your back with your arms resting at your sides, your legs bent at the knees and your feet flat on the ground.

Movement

Tighten your abdominals and slowly lift your hips off the floor into a bridge position, keeping your back straight.

Tip

Make sure to keep your trunk stiff throughout the exercise and your arms flat on the floor.

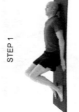

MEDBRIDGE   Disclaimer: This program provides exercises related to your condition that you can perform at home. As there is a risk of injury with any activity, use caution when performing exercises. If you experience any pain or discomfort, discontinue the exercises and contact your health care provider.

Login URL: www.medbridgego.com • Access Code: DY3ZJRFX • Date printed: 05/07/2021

Supine Pelvic Tilt

REPS: 20 | DAILY: 1 | WEEKLY: 4

Setup
Begin by lying on your back with your knees bent and feet resting on the floor.

Movement
Slowly tilt your pelvis forward, then tilt it back to neutral, and tilt it backward. Repeat these movements.

Tip
Make sure to concentrate your movements only on your pelvis.

STEP 1   STEP 2

Supine Pelvic Clock

REPS: 20 | DAILY: 1 | WEEKLY: 4

Setup
Begin lying on your back with legs bent and feet flat on the floor.

Movement
Imagine a clock lying flat on your pelvis with a ball at the center. Tilt your pelvis as if you were rolling the ball around the face of the clock in one direction. Then repeat in the other direction.

Tip
Make sure to keep your movements concentrated just on your pelvis. The rest of your back should be flat against the ground.

STEP 1   STEP 2

Supine 90/90 Alternating Toe Touch

REPS: 10 | DAILY: 1 | WEEKLY: 4

Setup
Lie on your back with your knees bent.

Movement
Lift your legs off the ground to form a 90 degree angle. Slowly lower one leg, touching your toes to the floor, then return to the starting position and repeat with the opposite leg.

Tip
Do not allow your low back to arch during the exercise.

STEP 1   STEP 2   STEP 3

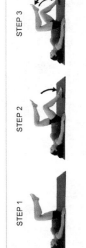

B. Wise Rehabilitation

Supine Diaphragmatic Breathing

MIN: 2-3 | DAILY: 1 | WEEKLY: 7

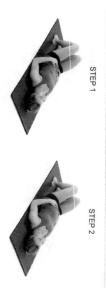

STEP 1　　STEP 2

Setup

Begin lying on your back with your knees bent and feet resting on the floor.

Movement

Exhale, drawing in your abdominals as if you are pulling your belly button toward the floor, then inhale, focusing on expanding your belly instead of your chest.

Tip

Make sure to keep your low back flat on the ground during the exercise.

Sidelying Thoracic Rotation with Open Book

REPS: 20 | DAILY: 1 | WEEKLY: 7

STEP 1　　STEP 2　　STEP 3

Setup

Begin lying on your side with your legs bent at a 75 degree angle and your arms together straight in front of you on the ground.

Movement

Slide your top hand back and forth over your bottom hand 5 times, rotating your shoulders. Then, lift your top arm straight up and over to the floor on your other side.

Tip

Make sure to keep your knees together and only rotate your back and upper arm. Your hips should stay facing forward.

Cat-Camel

REPS: 20 | DAILY: 1 | WEEKLY: 7

Setup

STEP 1　　STEP 2

Clinical Applications of CranioSacral Therapy

CST is well known for its multiple applications and positive results in thousands of cases like those of Mary Ellen and Onar. By facilitating and enhancing the body's self-corrective mechanisms, it has proved useful as both a primary and adjunctive treatment modality for a wide variety of dysfunctions, from coronary insufficiency to Crohn's disease.

The number of sessions required to achieve results depends on the complexity of the adaptive layers, patient defense mechanisms, and other factors. After an initial hands-on evaluation is conducted, a recommendation can be made. In general, if there is no change in condition after five or six sessions, CST may not be effective for that individual.

Following is a partial list of condition types that have shown response to CST in clinical applications. While research conducted at MSU proved the existence of the craniosacral system and its effect on health and disease, this information is based primarily on clinical observations over the last 15 years of practicing CST. Although no formal outcome studies have been conducted, thousands of patients have reported their results to us, and what is noted here are observations of clear and compelling results and trends.

Chronic Pain Syndromes

Arthritis: Degenerative and Inflammatory

CST enhances fluid motion, releases muscle tonus, and desensitizes facilitated segments, all of which contribute to joint rejuvenation. Excellent responses have been reported, including some results that have shown normalized blood studies.

Headache Syndromes

CST is excellent at identifying and treating a wide variety of underlying causes for headaches, including migraine, tension cephalalgia, fluid congestion, and hormonally related syndromes. Sutural immobility seems to be a contributing factor in migraines for many patients. CST addresses this problem, as well as autonomic and neuromusculoskeletal dysfunctions, both of which may be underlying causes of the migraine syndrome.

Pain Syndromes

All pain syndromes, including myofascial, neuromusculoskeletal, and radicular pain syndromes, have shown response to CST. Because of its effects on the autonomics, CST desensitizes facilitated segments and enhances fluid exchange throughout the body and psychoemotional effects. CST also addresses many of the neuromusculoskeletal, myofascial, and psychoemotional factors that may serve as contributing factors to chronic neck and back pain.

Reflexive Sympathetic Dystrophy

Reflexive sympathetic dystrophy (RSD) is a painful condition that results from the sympathetic nervous system going out of control. The cause could be an injury, entrapped nerve, inflammation, toxicity, or any circumstance that might feed an abnormal amount of energy into the sympathetic nervous system. Conservative medical treatment for this condition, which in extreme cases includes amputation of the painful area, has proven rather ineffective. The key to helping the RSD patient is discovering and resolving the underlying source of the excess energy. CST is well suited to finding and treating the underlying causes of RSD and subsequently resolving pain.

Spinal Dysfunctions

Spinal dysfunctions, including scoliosis, low-back (lumbar and lumbosacral) instability, disc compression, postoperative complications, and others, have shown response to CST. Once the underlying cause is determined, CST is effective in solving biomechanical, neurogenic, and facilitated segment problems.

Temporomandibular Joint Syndrome

Temporomandibular joint syndrome (TMJ) is a painful problem caused by the joints of the lower jaw becoming dysfunctional for any number of reasons. Surprisingly, TMJ can originate from a craniosacral system restriction that results in an imbalance between the temporal bones on each side of the head. Other causes include nervous tension that results in tooth grinding and/or jaw clenching, whiplash injury to the neck, or a malocclusion of the teeth. CST is highly effective at locating and alleviating the underlying problems. It is also highly effective at mobilizing temporal bones.

Traumatic Injuries

CST practitioners treat a multitude of traumatic brain and spinal cord injuries, including closed-head injuries, spinal cord injuries, whiplash and other spinal ligament strains, and nervous system sequelae due to injuries. Success varies, depending on the extent and severity of the injury. I usually do well with patients who suffer seizures subsequent to their head injuries, often eliminating the need for further medication. Although a small number of cases do not respond to CST, I have been treating seizure patients since 1975 and have yet to see an adverse reaction.

I have seen moderate improvement in the movement of paralyzed limbs due to head injuries. The greatest improvement usually appears in the area of intellect and social responsiveness. Some patients have had remarkable improvement in vision, hearing, smell, and taste, and in secondary autonomic dysfunction such as disequilibrium, cardiac pulmonary function, bowel function, urinary tract function, sexual function, and related conditions. The positive results are probably due to the effect of CST on the autonomics and related spinal cord segments, as well as its ability to reduce stress and anxiety.

Degenerative Diseases of the Central Nervous System

Until a few years ago it was thought that cerebrospinal fluid simply bathed the surface of the brain. All that changed with the use of radioactive tracers that flow with the fluid. It has since been observed that when tracers are injected into the ventricular system of the brain, they are distributed throughout the brain substance within minutes. Since cerebrospinal fluid carries all sorts of messenger molecules that facilitate communications between cells of different systems, it stands to reason that improving cerebrospinal fluid circulation may explain the success seen when CST is used to treat degenerative diseases such as Parkinson's disease.

Another recent discovery is that cerebrospinal fluid contains molecules that attach to metallic atoms that are deposited in the brain. These metallic atoms are then carried away and excreted from the body in a process known as *chelation*. Metal atoms deposited in the brain tissue are thought to be contributing factors in problems such as Alzheimer's disease and senility. Thus the improvement of cerebrospinal fluid circulation through CST may be considered preventive therapy.

Elderly patients who have trouble concentrating and putting words together have responded with increased mental alertness and brain function. By improving the circulation of blood, cerebrospinal fluid, and interstitial and intracellular fluid, CST helps clear toxic wastes accumulated in the brain cells and tissues.

Cerebrovascular Insufficiency Problems

CST has been shown to be effective in both preventing and recovering from stroke when thrombosis or arterial insufficiencies are causative agents. As soon as a patient's condition has stabilized after stroke and the danger of hemorrhage passes, CST can effectively help wash away toxic byproducts of blood cell deterioration to help enable a speedier recovery.

Postoperative Rehabilitation

CST is an excellent addition to any postsurgical rehabilitation program. It restores the movement of body fluids to areas traumatized by surgical procedures, which enhances the healing process and holds the potential for reducing the formation of adhesions and scar tissue. CST also helps remove residual toxicity of anesthetics and pain medications.

From about 1973 to 1974 I treated several postoperative neurological patients as early as the first postsurgical day with very good results. The neurosurgeon felt these patients demonstrated a decreased number of complications, lowered morbidity rates, and shortened recovery times. In general, the sooner the therapy begins, the better it is at helping to prevent complications.

Brain Dysfunctions

Autism

CST has shown great promise in cases of autism, a complex set of symptoms with no known origin. While it is not clear precisely which mechanisms are at work in either causing or "curing" the condition, it has been widely noted that patients generally inflict much less pain on themselves, display more affection toward others, and show improved social behavior after CST.

Cerebral Palsy

Cerebral palsy (CP) is a general term that means the brain is not working correctly. Because CST often has a positive effect on the motor control system, including relief of muscle spasticity, we do well with a majority of CP patients. There is occasional remarkable improvement, although sometimes there is little or no change. Either way it deserves a trial of approximately 10 sessions, although the rule holds true— the sooner we treat them the better these patients usually do. For example, if we treat a patient as an adolescent and can correct the underlying problem, the nerve pathways necessary for proper functioning may not be present because they never had a chance to form in the first place.

Learning Disabilities

I have treated a great number and variety of learning-disabled children. In my experience, over half of these children had problems with the craniosacral system. In cases like this, when the problem in the craniosacral system is resolved, the child has up to a 90% chance of overcoming his learning disabilities, especially in cases such as dyslexia and hyperkinesis. Quite often the disability simply disappears.

Motor System Problems

CST can almost invariably improve motor and speech problems. Even in the case of eye-motor problems, a skilled practitioner can tell in a matter of minutes if the problem is caused by tension in the membranes through which the nerves to the eyes pass. When this is the case, especially in children, the problem can often be permanently corrected in two or three sessions. Surgery for problems such as convergent strabismus (cross-eyes) can often be avoided. Patients treated with CST have also reported great success in cases of olfactory dysfunction and vertigo, although we have seen only moderate success with tinnitus.

Endocrine Disorders

Many endocrine disorders, including premenstrual tension, pituitary dysfunction, pineal gland problems, and related emotional problems, often respond favorably to CST. It enhances the mobilization of fluids and autonomic balancing, improves endocrine control, and relieves neuromusculoskeletal and psychoemotional symptoms. Releasing the dural sleeves that may be restricting nerve outflow to the adrenals, the thyroid, the spleen, the liver, the thymus, and the reproductive glands has also been very helpful in some patients.

Many Other Conditions

The most important thing to remember about CST is that it is extremely gentle and often resolves conditions in a shorter timeframe than many other approaches. Quite simply, it can almost always help in some fashion, even if simply to improve the chance of long-term success of other therapies used.

Contraindications of CranioSacral Therapy

Even in the most critical cases, CST has wide applications when used in conjunction with conventional treatment programs. However, the following are contraindications for the use of CST:[13]

1. *Acute intracranial hemorrhage:* Affecting the craniosacral system membranes may significantly change intracranial fluid pressure dynamics, which could interrupt the tenuous progress of clot formation and prolong the duration of the hemorrhage.

2. *Intracranial aneurysm:* Changing intracranial fluid pressure dynamics could potentially precipitate a leak or rupture of a dangerous, already present intracranial aneurysm.

3. *Recent skull fracture:* A very careful approach should be applied in the case of recent skull fracture, lest an increase in cranial bone motion leads to bleeding or a membranous tear.

4. *Herniation of the medulla oblongata:* A herniation of the medulla oblongata through the foramen magnum is a life-threatening situation. You would not want to alter fluid pressures within the craniosacral system by any means.

How to Learn CranioSacral Therapy

The Upledger Institute was developed in 1985 to educate the public and healthcare practitioners about the value of CST. Since that time, these techniques have been taught to more than 50,000 therapists in some 56 different countries.

Today the Upledger Institute is dedicated to teaching CST as it was originally developed. Its curriculum offers a full range of workshops totaling more than 500 hours of training.

In addition to providing a sound academic foundation, the training helps therapists develop the subtle senses of touch, motion, and energy perception necessary to become effective CST practitioners. The Upledger Institute also offers a two-level certification program to help ensure the quality of skills.

Because it was originally developed as a complementary modality for healthcare professionals, there is currently no single license to practice CST. Thanks to its rapid increase in practice and acceptance, however, plans are under way to create a separate and distinct professional license program.

Prospects for the Future

Over the last decade, positive clinical results and the public's growing acceptance of nontraditional healthcare methods have caused a surge in the demand for CST. It is continuing to become well known as an effective facilitator for the inherent healing processes with which every human being is endowed.

Its future in the field of rehabilitative care is bright. Yet its greatest value may be seen even earlier in the cycle of health: in the newborn nursery.[19] CST appears to be an efficient neutralizer for all types of birth traumas and their potential effects on the brain and spinal cord, including autonomic nervous function, endocrine function, and immune function. Research strongly suggests that the birth process alone may be responsible for numerous brain dysfunctions and central nervous system problems. CST carried out within the first few days of life could potentially reduce a wide variety of difficulties, many of which might not become apparent until later in life.

CST is also viewed as a successful method of integrating the body, mind, and spirit. This focus on "holistic" health may result in a significant reduction in disease and a great improvement in the quality of life.

References

1. Retzlaff EW et al: Nerve fibers and endings in cranial sutures research report, *J Am Osteopath Assoc* 77:474–475, 1978.

2. Retzlaff EW et al: Possible functional significance of cranial bone sutures, Report of the 88th session of the American Association of Anatomists, 1975.

3. Retzlaff EW et al: Structure of cranial bone sutures, research report, *J Am Osteopath Assoc* 75:607–608, 1976.

4. Retzlaff EW et al: Sutural collagenous [bundles] and their innervation in Saimiri Sciur[e]us, *Anat Rec* 187:692, 1977.

5. Retzlaff EW, Mitchell FL Jr: *The cranium and its sutures,* Berlin, 1987, Springer-Verlag.

6. Sperino G: *Anatomica humanica* 1:202–203, 1931.

7. Upledger JE: The reproducibility of craniosacral examination findings: a statistical analysis, *J Am Osteopath Assoc* 76:890–899, 1977.

8. Upledger JE: Relationship of craniosacral examination findings in grade school children with developmental problems, *J Am Osteopath Assoc* 77:760–776, 1978.

9. Woods JM, Woods RH: Physical findings related to psychiatric disorders, *J Am Osteopath Assoc* 60:988–993, 1961.

10. Upledger JE: Differences separate craniosacral therapy from cranial osteopathy, *Massage & Bodywork* X(4):20–22, 1995.

11. Upledger JE: Mechano-electric patterns during craniosacral osteopathic diagnosis and treatment, *J Am Osteopath Assoc* 1:49–50, 1979.

12. Upledger JE, Vredevoogd J: *CranioSacral Therapy,* Seattle, 1983, Eastland Press.

13. Upledger JE: *CranioSacral Therapy II: Beyond the Dura,* Seattle, 1987, Eastland Press.

14. Upledger JE: *SomatoEmotional Release and Beyond,* Berkeley, Calif, 1990, North Atlantic Books.

15. Lyttle J: An Olympian comeback, *Columbus Monthly* 1:105–107, 1996.

16. Murphy J: Olympic diver sinks vertigo with CranioSacral Therapy, *Adv Phys Therap* 7(42):5, 1996.

17. Bourne RA Jr: To Onar, with love, *Massage Ther J* 35(2):68–70, 72, 74, 1996.

18. Hammond F: The Upledger Institute offers Russian boy hope for more active life, *Nurse's Touch* 6(2):12, 1995.

19. Frymann VM: Relation of disturbances of craniosacral mechanisms to symptomatology of the newborn: a study of 1,250 infants, *J Am Osteopath Assoc* 65:1059, 1966.

What Is It?

DON ASH

As I travel around the country teaching I find the most frequently asked question is:

How do I first explain CranioSacral Therapy (CST) to my patients who have never heard of it before? I am a massage therapist; how do I tell someone I also do CST?

Tell your patients, "Hey I've learned a new technique that may help you in addition to our regular (massage, PT, OT, Chiropractic, etc.) session. Would you like to try it?"

The patient may ask, "Well, what is it?" My lesson from many sessions is in the frequent times patients have asked me to explain, prompting me to create the explanation I'll share with you now.

This is what I tell them: "Everyone has several kinds of rhythms in their body. There is the cardiac rhythm, in which the heart beats 60–80 times per minute. Then there is the respiratory rhythm of your breathing, in which you inhale and exhale 15–20 times per minute. Underneath those rhythms is another one called the CranioSacral Rhythm (CSR). In this rhythm your head gently expands and narrows and your spine gently lengthens and shortens in an effort to exchange and circulate cerebrospinal fluid. It does this 6–12 cycles per minute. The membranes that surround your head and spine act as a little hydraulic pump that draws this clear fluid out of your blood, bathes the brain

Reprinted with permission from Don Ash, *Lessons from the Sessions: Reflections of Journeys in CranioSacral Therapy* (Odyssey Press, 22 Nadeau Drive, P.O. Box 7307, Gonic, NH 03839-7307), 19–23.

and spinal cord with it, and then returns it to the blood supply. In this way the cerebrospinal fluid is filtered and renewed. It is important fluid because it supplies nutrients, carries away waste products, and acts as a fluid protective covering for the brain and spinal cord.

"The cardiac rhythm can be felt at the neck, wrist, and ankles. The rhythm of the lungs can be felt at the shoulders, neck, chest, and belly. Like these other rhythms, the CranioSacral Rhythm can be felt from all over the body—the legs, pelvis, sacrum, shoulders, and head.

"If I were to hold your ribs and resist your lungs from expanding, you would move to allow your lungs freedom to continue their rhythm. What we do in CranioSacral Therapy is *very gently* hold the rhythm and watch as the body gently moves to free itself. As it does this, releases occur and restrictions in the body change. Just as bruised ribs from a fall might keep you from breathing properly, a fall on your tailbone or a bump on the head may keep your beautiful craniosacral system from working properly.

"So we gently hold and wait for releases. Releases occur in the form of heat, pulsing, muscle twitching. Sometimes the eyes may blink or gurgling sounds occur in the digestive system. You may feel part of your body soften, or gently shift and spread. Breathing patterns may change. A deep feeling of relaxation is a common reaction to treatment."

Some releases are gentle, but sudden. I offer this analogy as an example: "Have you ever come home from a hard day and said to yourself, oh boy, am I tired, I can't wait to go to sleep tonight? So you get into your bed, the room is dark, and the house is quiet; you can feel sleep overcoming you. Your eyes get heavy and just start to close—and surprise!!!!!! Your body jumps. Has that ever happened to you?" Ninety-eight percent of patients nod their head yes to this. I continue, "The other thing that can sometimes happen with this work is that your body may get very still before or during the release process. It's a special point because it is a Significance Detector for your body. Some-times as your body is resting here on the air mattress and my hands are listening to the rhythm of your craniosacral system, your body might move into the position it was in when you got hurt. This often happens with people having pain and dysfunction from slips, falls, motor vehicle accidents, and traumatic events such as being beaten up in a fight. Your rhythm automatically stops, and releases begin to occur. You enter a point of stillness we call a Significance Detector because the position the body moves into, or what you are thinking, is often an important (significant) part of the healing and letting go process."

Sometimes there are emotions held in the body that are a part of the release process. I once had a patient who could not remember what had happened after being in a single-car accident. She was a single mother caring for two young children. She was in a lot of pain, unhappy, and concerned because her pain and limited range of motion in her neck and arms had gone on for over a year. She was fearful she would be unable to continue to care for her children.

She had been to conventional therapies such as PT, OT, Chiropractic, and had been seen by orthopedists and neurologists. Nothing seemed to help.

When she came to me I explained to her about CranioSacral Therapy, and the cranial rhythm. I also told her about releases and allowing the body to release what it will. I asked her to lie down on her back and I began to listen to her rhythm at her feet, then her thighs, then her pelvis. At the pelvic diaphragm, she gently turned and curled up into the fetal position, closed her eyes, and said her ankles, wrists, shoulders, and neck hurt. She said she could see the color red. She then began to cry. Her rhythm had stopped.

I kept my hands in the pelvic diaphragm position, with the patient still on her side. I told her these were emotional and physical memories held in her body that were releasing and if she could stay with this process for a few minutes it would be helpful. She was able to stay with the process for five or six minutes and then she stopped crying, straightened out on the table, and sat up.

She said, "You know, now I can remember the accident." She explained in detail that she didn't see the black ice and she felt the car start to skid. "I saw the telephone pole coming towards me and I tried to press hard on the pedals; my feet went under the pedals. I straightened my arms out with a strong grip on the steering wheel and I remember being so scared and thinking about who would care for my children and what would happen to them. When the crash came I felt pain in my ankles, wrists, and shoulders. I felt my neck snap and the last thing I saw just before I blacked out was the red hood of my car crashing through the windshield."

She then tried to turn her neck and exclaimed, "Wow, I can turn my neck and I don't have pain. What just happened?" I explained about still points and Significance Detectors. That is to say, her body moved into the position it needed, in order to release the effects of the trauma from the motor vehicle accident. It also provided her with a SomatoEmotional Release (SER), releasing an emotional charge that accompanied the trauma at the moment of impact and immediately after.

She came in twice after that session for massage and exercise, and then I discharged her to return to family life pain free.

So, CranioSacral Therapy is a gentle method of listening to the body and encouraging change. It is using very light touch (5 grams) to encourage releases that may include heat, pulsing, gurgling of the digestive tract, muscle movements, and breath change. Releases may be emotional, in the form of tears, laughter, and/or memories—that may produce feelings of fear, shame, sadness, anger, remorse—that also can come to the patient's awareness and thereby release.

The most important part about CST, and a real lesson from every session, is that the body will lead the way, and do what the patient needs—and do what the therapist is able to help facilitate. Therefore, massage therapists, PTs, OTs—those practitioners who want to work with the physical body—will do that (facilitate), and experience, by and large, all physical releases (heat, pulsing, etc.). Those therapists who feel confident in assisting with emotional release usually invest a lot of time and energy training in SomatoEmotional Release and may facilitate that event for the patient. The body is able to recognize the level of work the therapist is able to facilitate.

After a short discussion with the patient covering some of the elements I've mentioned, I ask if it sounds like something they would like to try. They usually say yes and away we go on our adventure.

An Historical Introduction to Craniosacral Therapy

RICHARD GROSSINGER

Definition

Craniosacral therapy (CST) is a technique for tapping into the body's many layers and matrices, using educated hands to sense and adjust tensions of fascia and viscera and subtle pressures of fluids, revitalizing organs and restoring underlying rhythms toward their natural states. It is also a paraphysical art using light but intentional touch to transduce mind, matter, and energy into one another. I think of it as a fusion of a mild, noninvasive surgery—more delicate than any massage—with a wordless psychoanalysis whereby palpation releases cysts of trapped emotional and somatic energy.

With other osteopathic disciplines like Polarity, Visceral Manipulation, Zero Balancing, and Myofascial Release, CST is the forerunner of a post-technological healing that parallels quantum physics in its capacity to weigh virtually imperceptible cellular vectors, use mindedness and breath to track and influence tissue systems and metabolic processes, and translate probabilistic and hypothetical events into real ones. At that level it is a relativistic system that entertains paradoxical, even contradictory, possibilities at the same time.

Note: This piece is a combined abridged excerpt from a number of the author's books. Most of it comes from *Planet Medicine: Modalities;* smaller sections were taken from *Embryogenesis: Species, Gender, and Identity; Embryos, Galaxies, Sentient Beings: How the Universe Makes Life;* and *The Bardo of Waking Life.*

Origins in Osteopathy

Osteopathic medicine, the field out of which CST matriculated, is a legacy of the pre-technological epoch when palpating tissues was the primary scientific mode of diagnosing and treating health and disease, hence a revival of an original mechanical medicine practiced with a million variants by cultures ranging from African and South American tribes to island peoples of the Pacific and folk doctors of Europe. Most Third and Fourth World villages and cities still possess remarkable native manipulators and bonesetters practicing crafts passed from generation to generation. They have no written tradition, no formal school, no medical theory, and no cross-cultural contact with one another.

Manual medicine has a long and distinguished Western history. Pre-osteopathic folk traditions of "trampling in the fields," "weighing salt," and "the shepherd's hug"—simple somatic techniques—hearken back to Neolithic and probably Palaeolithic times. Andrew Still's later "invention" of osteopathy as a system and Daniel Palmer's chiropractic variation were revivals of traditional European bonesetting and healing touch. Still systematized them according to principles of intellectual anatomy and physics and provided an arena for their fusion with modern technological medicine (allopathy).

Early osteopathy interpreted the body as a dense geometric grid supported by a skeleton, activated by nerves, and permeated with channels flushed by systolic and diastolic motion. Trained academically as an engineer, Still could not help but initially view the organism as another dynamic system, one that occasionally developed congestions and blocks. He made corrections based on his intuition of mechanical relationships among its parts (i.e., bones, fascia, circulations of fluids). The son of a doctor, he had attempted allopathy and had given up on it.

"I was born and raised to respect and confide in the remedial power of drugs, but after many years of practice in close conformity to the dictation of the very best medical authors and in consultation with representatives of the various schools, I failed to get from drugs the results hoped for and I was face to face with the evidence that medicine was not only untrustworthy but dangerous.

"The mechanical principles on which osteopathy is based are as old as the universe. I discovered them while I was in Kansas. . . .

"As I was an educated engineer of five years' schooling I began to look at the human framework as a machine. . . . I began to experiment with man's body as a master mechanic would when he had in his charge any machinery which needed to be kept perfectly adjusted and in line in order to get perfect work. There are many ways by which a machine may be adjusted. An osteopathic operator is not expected to depend on any one method or manipulation for the adjustment of a bone."[1]

During the 1870s Still cultivated modes of treatment based on ever more subtle analyses of anatomical relationships. "We, as engineers, have but one question to ask," he asserted: "What has the body failed to do?"[2]

Although there was no consistent formula to Still's techniques, he did generally use pressure and adjustment to restore blood supply and nerve responsiveness in afflicted areas; he worked from the perspective that natural flow would lead to the organs' reestablishing their original dynamic relationships and harmonics. He did not have to try to antidote every germ and flush out every toxin because a kinetic system regaining its own efficiency would accomplish all that without further toxic interference.

His mechanical treatments are models of ingenuity, and they were responsible for much of osteopathy's early success. For instance, he pinpointed pneumonia as a constriction of the thoracic/pulmonary system leading to stagnation of the venous system and impure blood, curable through sequential adjustments of different bones. In the case of a cataract of the eye, he advised:

"Adjust the bones of the upper spine, ribs and neck and re-establish normal nerve and blood supply. Then make a gentle tapping of the eye to loosen the crystalline lens a little. With one finger give a few flips or gentle taps on the back of another finger the soft part of which is held against the side of the eye. This tapping should be just strong enough to make the eye ache a little. Without any surgical interference whatever I have been rewarded in a majority of cases by the disappearance of that white substance in the eye called a cataract."[3]

Insofar as the critical kinetic junctions among bones, muscles, and nerves are more or less obvious, there is no reason to question the potential effectiveness of osteopathy in the treatment of injuries, strains, sciatica, or even constipation. In this use osteopathy is no more or less than an expanded version of therapeutic massage or even maternal caregiving. But Still enlarged his system to address diabetes, mumps, hysteria, alcoholism, and mental disease. Even though he also employed pharmacy, diet, hygiene, surgery, and verbal therapy, his emphasis was primarily on understanding and reorganizing anatomy, not only in the gross sense but at ever subtler levels of hormonal and fascial microanatomy until he had mastered the entire anatomicophysiological mechanism.

The initial prejudice is to think that osteopathy cannot be the same as medicine or as therapeutic because it lacks tools, refuses intellectual categories, and utilizes mere mechanical and skeletal adjustment or visceral massage—as though to palpate the intestinal region could cure a tumour as effectively as to cut into the very tissue.

But if we view the osteopathic principles from a different perspective, we can see that osteopathy is also a complex and complete medicine. It proposes treatments based as much on mechanical cause and effect as allopathy, though it translates the burden of mechanical correction to the already functioning organism, which is viewed as perfect.

Osteopathy doesn't need heavy equipment because it relies on the viscera to respond self-curatively to a quantum of energy directed appropriately in the right spot. Allopathy, with its more entropic view of the universe, takes account of the grand array of parasites, germs, viruses, bacteria, toxins, malignancies, and "bad" genes and assumes constant remedial work is needed for each of us even to survive. In a sense, modern medicine boggles itself with the complexity of the universe to such a degree that diagnosing and correcting defects become substitutes for living. Osteopathy, by contrast, assumes that most pathologies can be reversed by simple mechanical stimulation or manipulation, that the body is already working well enough to solve most of its problems but will respond favorably to a sensitively directed adjustment.

Osteopathy premises that we are self-organized primarily at the level of interrelationships of bones, fluids, and viscera. Thus, it considers most of the synthetic chemical, radiational, genetic, and surgical modalities invasive, for they undermine an ontologically prior level of function and self-healing and seek to penetrate, according to a purely conceptual and idealized paradigm, the molecular realm where disease products supposedly originate and spread.

By the allopathic line of reasoning, molecular and even atomic technologies must one day take over tracking the origin of all diseases and curing those that can be cured. But what if none of this is possible, efficient, or even necessary? What if the molecular and atomic realms are *not* the functional dimension of life? What if these contain mere subsidiary effects of cofactors originating elsewhere? What if creatures have all the requirements for health fully and holistically integrated at a tissue level? What if the cohesive synergy of cells is the sole active psychosomatic level of life?

After all, we do not actually understand the underlying principle that links cells together and induces them to conduct chemical cycles and metabolism functionally.

By this line of reasoning, osteopathy is not only directly medical but in some ways more medical than surgery. Far from being superficial, its touch is exquisite, as the physician works his way into the patient's system by assessing complex reciprocal forces, stacking lines of tension and immobility, meeting and incrementalizing tissue resistance, and following sensations and distortions to their exact sources in organs. What could be more empirical? Who established a rule that you have proximally to contact and incise actual disease products in order to heal tissues? If actual illnesses are the consequence of deeper imbalances rather than the source of the diseases they give names to, then orthodox medicine would be regularly attacking the effects of pathology rather than its causes. It would be invading nonlinear homeostatic systems along one-dimensional vectors.

Insofar as manual practitioners treat serious visceral diseases and psychopathologies, they do not regard their techniques as merely musculoskeletal (engineering-based); they view palpation as a means of accessing the core mechanism of life.

Still himself came to endow the kinetic life system with almost magical properties. He perceived that the circulation of fluids, energy, and substances through the body was so subtle and highly complex that it occurred on many levels simultaneously, including arterial, venous, nervous, lymphatic, and cerebrospinal components. What he could not explicitly assign to a level of circulation, he assigned to the collective circulatory mechanism. Beginning as an ardent materialist, he ended up describing the lungs as "organs, beings or personalities of life . . . the functions of the heart . . . imparting life and knowledge to the blood."[4]

Osteopathy to this day embraces a profound original contradiction. It is, on the one hand, a quasi-academic medicine much like allopathy, and on the other, a new paradigm in body-mind relations and complexity-based life dynamics. It would appear that Still, while proposing mechanical and material precepts, inadvertently discovered another system and, without realizing it, tapped into the organizing life current.

There are historical precedents: Samuel Hahnemann stumbled upon homeopathy's energetic microdoses because he did not realize that high molecular dilutions were chemically inert; thus, he applied them medicinally *as if they were* elevated potencies of matter and ascribed dynamic effects to them. Still entered a realm of mysterious visceral energy by not understanding that his mechanical model was merely the entry point into the complexity of organized cells. While stacking weights and densities of tissues and balancing fascia, he invented a system for conducting energies within living fields of bones and tissues. Osteopathy, which began as physics-like equations of mass and surgery-like manipulations, spawned vitalistic techniques. Once healers experienced and followed the resonance of myriad currents of "Liquid Light," they found themselves inside the vital principle, handling life itself.

Cranial Osteopathy

Palpation as energy medicine owes a good part of its development to William G. Sutherland. A student at Still's College of Osteopathy in Kirksville, Missouri, Sutherland was familiar with the school's famous mounted disarticulated skull—a specimen in which the individual cranial bones were pulled apart and wired into positions true to their original structure yet revealing the complexity of their sutures. In 1899, "glancing at the Beauchene skull, he became transfixed by the squamosal suture of the temporal bones, the rolling-overlap joint between temporals and parietals. The words 'Bevelled like the gills of a fish, and indicating articular mobility for a respiratory mechanism' flashed into his mind."[5]

At the time, even among osteopaths, the cranium was presumed to be a fixed, interlocked dome (to this day there is no clear recognition of the pliability of the bones of the skull in most American medical texts).

It was not until his fifth year of practice in Minnesota that Sutherland got to explore his intuition. He purchased a football helmet, small pieces of India rubber, leather, straps, shoemaker's buckles, and sewing materials and turned the helmet into a device for restricting the individual bones of skull and thus testing their ranges of motion. That is, he further immobilized his own supposedly immobile bones and, to the distress of his wife, induced an astonishing array of mental and internal ailments. When naturally occurring, these symptoms would lend themselves to cure through cranial manipulation.

Taking his cues from his own sensations of restraint, Sutherland explored the sinuous and minute cycles of motility among the many tiny articulated bones; he painstakingly remapped the cranial skeleton as dynamic tissue. Then he developed a variety of means for manipulating and balancing the skull's individual zones, always with precision because of the subtle properties of such miniscule fields of articulation. He soon built a practice based on treating a variety of emotional and physical disorders, including migraines and various emotional maladies, all through cranial osteopathy.

Sutherland was curious to find out what happened when he tied down all the straps at once. In this uncomfortable headlock (which, all the same, should have been entirely static from the standpoint of most medical theories) he was astonished to feel his sacrum begin to oscillate rhythmically while becoming warmer. He had penetrated what was to become the "core link" of cranial osteopathy, the energetic and mechanical conjugation between the occiput and the sacrum through the supple spinal dura.

"[Sutherland] told of lying down, his head in the V-shape head rest; of imposing compression by gradual tension of buckle and strap." He described the excitations he had experienced as he approached near-unconsciousness. . . : "'A sensation of warmth followed,'" he explained. "'And also a remarkable movement of fluid up and down the spinal column, throughout the ventricles. . . . Fantastic!'"[6]

He eventually developed a phenomenological anatomy based on craniosacral hydraulics. Ultimately he came to rediscover the body as a relativistic, fluid form, combining respiratory, circulatory, skeletal, emotional, and other properties in a series of interrelated ripples and vibrations. The cranial rhythm flows as a deep, long tide with sub-tides and wavelets inside it, conducting it and also radiating from it. The long tide forms the central vortex of the body, maintaining its biodynamic equilibrium. This grounds the power of hydraulic palpation. The separate subwaves and wavelets continue to assimilate unresolved experiences and autonomic functions within the central nervous system.

The crises and energies of tissues and the unconscious impressions of living creatures imprint themselves from the cells and nervous system in the cerebrospinal fluid to be cleansed and transmuted. Palpation enhances this process, thus evoking the deepest autonomic, embryogenic elements of biological existence.

The craniosacral modality was later named for the cranium and sacrum through which this current under membrane and tissue is most directly accessed. However, craniosacral therapy is bodywide and not limited to the hydraulic core. A common mistake is to assume that the process has primarily to do with conditions of the cranial, spinal and sacral skeleton and the movements of its bones. The rhythm is in fact a component of and guide to events within the whole organism—its viscera, psyche, and even its etheric fields.

The modern development of cranial osteopathy since Sutherland emphasizes riding the tide: light over heavy adjustments, tissue dialogue over mechanical movement, and psychospiritual integration over structural repair. It is still a manual medicine based in thermodynamics—informed touch is the starting point for all procedures—but it has also become a holistic modality.

The combination of Still's and Sutherland's techniques has led to a post-modern medical system. Probably the most significant single factor in its advance has been the shift of focus from musculoskeletal modalities to visceral and craniosacral ones. As contemporary osteopath Rollin E. Becker wrote to Sutherland in 1949:

"The more I study Osteopathy, the more it seems to boil down to a Highly Intelligent fluid surrounded and held in shape by fascial membranes.

"Allow the fascial strains to correct what might be present, allow the fluid to resume its normal TIDAL mechanism, and all associated pathologies in the muscle, skin, blood vessels or nerves will correct themselves. Bend to the oar through the fascia, and ride the TIDE to the shore by way of the fluid."[7]

Cranial Osteopathy and Embryology

The prime—in fact, the only—capacity medicine has is to hitch itself to the embryogenic process, the "inner physician." If a single cell contains the whole plan of an organism and a mechanism for enacting it, how can an exterior physician rival or replicate this? He can assist it, catalyze its sluggishnesses, and attempt to remove more blatant impediments in its way, but he cannot sculpt or congeal anything resembling a lump of protoplasm let alone a breathing, conscious, philosophizing organ. Thus, medicine archetypally is meant to awaken the totems that lie at the heart of development, to encourage their miracles to go on happening.

From its implicit (experiential) comprehension of self-organizing life fields, quantum density, decoherence spin networks, and tensegrity of cytoskeletons, osteopathic palpation is no longer limited (at best) to possibilities of manipulating proximate and contingent tissue; it is now considered plausible to attempt to change cell shape, structure, relationship, and even heredity by activating a range of morphogenetically inductive factors. Cranial and energetic disciplines have thus been legitimated to explore the entire universe of soma, psyche, health, and disease as a relativistic, post-cybernetic modality. The fusion of touch, intention, and energy-channeling portends a possible medical science of indeterminate scope and breadth.

Today's quantum palpation was not something that Still could specify from a nineteenth-century theocratic perspective that understood physical energy only nonmolecularly and nonholographically. He was an engineer. He construed the organism as a machine of flesh and bones. His strategies for repairing that machine originated in familiar technological metaphors. He did not anticipate the transformation of body architectures into resonant and scalar waves or thermodynamics going past quantum uncertainty limits into autonomous phase states.

Yet once Still (and his followers) began grabbing bones and fascia by their protrusions, following their tissue resistance, and draining energy like a sponge, they entered into the unfathomed realm of the body's reciprocities, dimensionalities, transition fields, and the subtle impregnation of mind in organs. They were dealing with a machine perhaps, but it was a trans-cybernetic, nonergodic machine of an order that had not yet been imagined.

The original physical projections of Still keep providing osteopathy with an empirical anatomical basis. This is therapeutically critical, for intuitively palpated energy forms occupy the same spaces as concrete tissue structures, and informed diagnosis and treatment must acknowledge the actual densities and shapes of organs.

Even if it is possible that all of the functions of the body are reducible to fulcra, levers, pulleys, and pumps, the living anatomicochemical mechanism functions as extremely complex gradations of kinetic energy between gross and subtle levels, with motion and potential constantly flowing downwards from the skeleton to the cytoskeleton and upwards from the molecular nucleus to the neuroviscera. Cells and molecules, after all, also have tiny fulcra, pulleys, pumps, etc. The overall machinery of the body is multidimensional, nano-mechanical, kinesthetic, and phenomenological, and within the domain of mind, it fluctuates as surely as photons between waves and particles.

Still set a living machine in motion. Yet, no matter how the operator/practitioner behaves, the machine can never be run as an assembly-line robot. Receptive and sentient in every aspect, it takes vectors imposed onto it and transposes them into other vectors which generate yet others.

Matter also generates energy, especially in living tissue. It resonates with its own emergent waves of sentience.

What Still did not fully perceive was that the force he directed into the body from the premise of a machinery was received by that machinery as nonlinear impulses and hologrammatic currents. The same was true for Sutherland; his (albeit delicate) clockwork of cranial osteopathy was also a transfusion of energy of an indeterminate nature.

The original machine has not been discarded; it continues to occupy space with its exquisite architectures, to translate simple into complex energy. But it is the kind of machine that, once it perceives the mind of a therapeutic conductor, leads him transpersonally into its own plan.

Today osteopathy is both a manipulative medicine seeking legitimacy under the blanket of professional health care and supporting manual medical trainings that mirror conventional ones, and an innovative paraphysical science tracking quantum currents in fabrics and fields. It has become, for many, a mode of placing hands through skin on bones and viscera and touching the soul.

Craniosacral Therapy

Although many have contributed to the revival of Sutherland's science, it was primarily a medical osteopath, John Upledger, who had the ingenuity to reinvent cranial osteopathy as CranioSacral Therapy in the late 1970s while he was part of an interdisciplinary team of doctors and physical and biological scientists at Michigan State University. During a surgery he noticed the movement of the dura mater membrane—an inexplicable pulse that was synchronous with neither the breath nor the heart rate. He observed the pulse's regularity, intensity, and centrality (he was trying to hold the dural membrane still for plaque removal by using two sets of forceps, but its pulsing movement prevailed against his mechanical pressure). He later verified these findings clinically and in extensive autopsies.

The craniosacral rhythm is a fundamental pulse like breath and heartbeat, though quieter and less metabolism-driven than the rush of either blood or air. Upledger extrapolated a pressure-stat system with the compressive flow of cerebrospinal fluid providing its engine. From there he began developing means of diagnosis and treatment based on dynamics arising from system and trademarked his method as "Cranio-Sacral Therapy" (and later, "SomatoEmotional Release") to distinguish it from the more heavy-handed thrusting manipulation common in the osteopathic trade and also from post-Freudian bioenergetics.

In defiance of both medical and osteopathic establishments, he taught a widening compass of manual techniques to lay people in hopes of increasing the base of qualified healers and practitioners in the world. Thus, cranial osteopathy evolved into craniosacral therapy or, more precisely, Upledger adapted and transformed many aspects of Sutherland's system into a new cranial medicine, retaining techniques, reinterpreting techniques, developing new techniques, and combining elements in innovative ways based on empirical discoveries.

Upledger describes the craniosacral system as being made up of "the three-layered membrane system that we call the meninges, ... the cerebrospinal fluid enclosed by this membrane system, ... and the structures within the membrane system which control fluid input and outflow for the system."[8] As a result of the absorption and extraction of cerebrospinal fluid, the full range of bones, tissues, fascia, and viscera— from cranium to phalanges, along the spine and outward—participate in the aforementioned cycle of flexion (inward curling) and extension (outward unfurling).

The cerebrospinal network is the internal milieu for the suffusion of all the fluids and innervations of the brain and nervous system into the muscles and viscera. Because the hydrostatic cycle encompasses the brain, spinal cord, and pituitary and pineal glands, it has far-reaching effects on the body's functions. Its pumping action integrates with musculoskeletal, vascular, lymphatic, and neuroendocrine processes. Dysfunctions and pathologies in any local region will reflect along cross-binding angles and axes multidimensionally in the whole organism.

Craniosacral treatments are rooted in and tracked through the requirements and manifestations of the bodywide hydraulic network driven by the pressure of the cerebrospinal fluid (as more of it is produced by the choroid plexuses within the ventricles of the brain than is reabsorbed by the arachnoid bodies).

The craniosacral flexion-extension cycle extending down the dural tube to the viscera is likely generated and perpetuated because the dura-mater membrane is almost completely impermeable to the cerebrospinal fluid. Within this membrane, a homeostasis develops, regulating and rebalancing forces that build and release pressure. The craniosacral therapist, palpating and tractioning the differential pressures of this system, changes visceral hydraulics and chemistry.

The bones of the cranium, proximate to the reigning functions of the nervous system, tend to translate distortion downhill (along the spine and its dural membrane secondarily, and then through fascia, tendons, and ligaments). Sites for initiating therapy include the dura mater attached like handles to the bones of the skull, the temporomandibular joint through the tentorium cerebelli, the muscular component of the xiphoid process of the sternum, and the pelvic and urogenital diaphragms and their muscles and fascia.

Cranial components like the sphenoid bone (which lies mostly behind the eyes and nose), the falxes cerebri and cerebelli, the occipital, parietal, and temporal bones, etc., function as levers, valves, and pistons of this system. The sphenoid—butterfly in shape and possibly homologous to the pelvis at the other end of the spine—is accessible to palpation only at the outer tips of the eye sockets; it is adjusted by light compression, decompression, twisting, and sliding to alter other components of the face and skull and thereby transpose freedom of movement downward. The temporal bones can be set in traction by a firm, gentle pulling of the external ear lobes. Other components of the system may be accessed from inside the mouth through the teeth or hard palate or from a remote stimulation of the dural membrane itself.

A web of connective tissue intertwines and interpenetrates all the viscera from the meninges of the brain, down the front and back of the body, all the way to the bottoms of the feet. Fascia encompasses the musculature of the shoulders, chest, back of the ribs, dural tube, and pelvis as well as the wrappings of the entirety of organs and limbs (pericardium, intestines, genitals, etc.) in what is essentially a dynamically complex but single sheet. Its cohesive plait provides pathways for palpating stress lines and tracking them to impacted sites, likewise for unraveling the knots.

The fascial web develops in an indivisible piece out of mesodermal tissue and envelops the entire body. Its global expanse, heterogenous penetration of tissue, and activation by the cerebrospinal pulse through the nervous system allow it to transmit and receive the cranial rhythm everywhere. A single system embryogenically, the fabric of fascia interpenetrates itself and all the organs. From the falx cerebri to the tentorium cerebelli down the internal lining of the occiput to the carotid foramen of the temporal bone winds one dynamic sheet. With a change in scale and orientation, that sheet continues to the pericardium in the thorax and the respiratory diaphragm; from there, with another change in vector and scale, to the psoas muscle, pelvis, corpora cavernosa of the penis and clitoris, legs, and bottoms of the feet. The fascia functions as both a map and highway through the body—a natural neural, mechanical, and hydraulic medium for the transmission of palpatory remedies.

In the words of Upledger and his co-author Jon D. Vredevoogd, the body fascia are "a slightly mobile, continuous from head-to-toe, laminated sheath of connective tissue which invests in pockets (between lamina) of all of the somatic and visceral structures of the body. . . . By direct connections and common osseous anchorings, the extradural fascia and the meninges are interrelated and interdependent in terms of their motion. Therefore, the amount of diagnostic and prognostic information which can be obtained from the examination of fascial mobility or restriction is limited only by the palpatory skill and anatomical knowledge of the examiner. Attention is directed to the rate, amplitude, symmetry and quality of the craniosacral motion and its reflection throughout the body."[9]

Craniosacral Techniques

The palpator picks a spot for entry and, meeting tissue resistance, adds about five more grams of force to mobilize not the dermis or pure musculature but the total energetic pattern issuing from that point. The amount of force may seem like more than five grams because of meeting tissue resistance before adding any quanta of pressure.

The touch is the lightest possible because it must be durable; it must travel deep into viscera, honing toward core without attaching to intermediate structures and dissipating itself there. Too firm a touch immediately activates connective-tissue resistance; the palpation then becomes conventional massage. Once the touch becomes too heavy, the organism begins to respond less on the level of craniosacral or visceral sensitivity and more in terms of neuromuscular tension and stress patterns. This is not like going from good to bad; it is switching therapeutic modes (and is rarely successful).

A good rule of thumb for a therapist is: have the touch be as light as you can bear, i.e., as light as you can impose while still imagining you are making contact and doing something, as light as you can discern and palpably differentiate—and then go a hair lighter.

Listening itself can be more therapeutic than actively adjusting because "just listening" does also adjust, very subtly. Usually when you think you are doing nothing—right on the cusp of active intention—is when you are most receptive, least intrusive, and most profoundly engage with deep organic structure. When one breaks with listening to act willfully on tissue, listening may stop and the palpation may become shallower, as the hands cease to melt into tissue layers and follow their torque—and the organs resist.

Even medium touch can be coopted by and fuse with an "irrelevant" tissue layer that happens to get in the way. The healer must instead gather up stress lines one by one, a vector at a time, somewhat like following ripples to a center from which they radiate, stacking them as she goes. Too light a touch merely distorts the ripples; too heavy a hand plows right through them.

In working with fascia, viscera themselves, or the craniosacral rhythm, the therapist circumscribes a part of the body with both hands, perhaps one on the lower back, one on the belly. He then adds pressure with the top hand until he feels the tissues start to move. The hand senses out the contour and directional orientation of muscle fibers and fascia and palpates in a shear, torquing, or rotary motion; its direction anterior-posterior, longitudinal-transverse, or multi-angular and oblique. Gradually the region relaxes and reorients; its tissues soften; then the pressure is released and a new motion may be initiated, either there or elsewhere, depending on the resulting stasis.

The stress lines are little beads that fall along different trajectories and in slightly different planes. Gathering them is a bit like trying to balance an increasingly higher tower of little paper boxes not resting flush atop one another, except that the skilled palpator's juggling is supported by the tissues' guiding grains, their intrinsic pliability and density, and also by almost indescribable currents of energy.

As the body responds to induction, it guides the hand along the path of the blockage to where tissue has been restricted and rigidified and "wants" to be released. It has semi-rotated, sidebent, and corkscrewed in some combination to shorten its ranges of movement and reduce the shearing and compression effects at specific nodes, and it has likely developed adhesions and barriers to motility with adjacent organs. By gently accreting lines of force and balancing multiple reciprocal axes in all three (or four) dimensions, the therapist untangles and liberates restrictions and adhesions layer by layer, gathering residual energy and mass in the process and continuing inward to other nodes.

Since most organs are blocked from direct therapist access by musculoskeletal structures and other organs, continued light stacking and balancing is needed to follow a vector far enough in to reach, for instance, the pancreas, spleen, stomach, kidneys, ureter, structures inside the skull or behind the eyes, etc. Sometimes the therapist may raise, fold, or torque the body across the pelvis, shoulders, or chest to produce a tauter path to the proper site at the most appropriate therapeutic angle and depth. Clearly this is a method requiring great anatomical dexterity, hair-trigger sensitivity, and delicacy in stacking planes and pressures and pulling vectors.

The goal is to disencumber these areas through (mostly) indirect techniques, that is, by stimulation of intrinsic rhythms or even exaggeration and support of a dysfunctional pattern until it swings so far to its distortedly favored side that it returns naturally to the other limit (restoration by going with rather than fighting a distortion is a standard osteopathic technique).

Often the therapist finds the right level of force and depth by ever so subtly adding and removing increments of weight to her hand while fine-tuning the angle of entry with minute rotations at her wrist and shoulder. The former allows finer adjustments, the latter grosser ones. The tissue may lead the hand in a circular trajectory. The therapist tries to find the line of untangling, i.e., where there is a slightly greater centrifugal force, and makes a stand there. She gently stops the circle and slowly steers its orbit into the angular force, a sensation which is simultaneously like pulling taffy, attracting metal filings with a small magnet, and pulling tight a drawstring from far away. Gathering any slack remaining in the drawstring, she continues to resist the old orbit and to reign in (as she senses them) even tinier loops of slack.

Cumulatively the slack represents distances within the body. As it is imaginarily drawn in, the hand is influencing either more interior organs or tissues further away. For instance, entry and steering at the level of the bladder can pull "strings" along the ureter or down to the bottom of the foot. At the same time, the therapist tracks globally, picking up any resonance or vibration from outside her primary trajectory and allowing her touch to ride the waves of cerebrospinal fluid expressed by flexion and extension of the whole system. The larger rhythms guide the treatment to new sites or lines of entry.

The motion is followed to differing degrees with both hands until it stops (this is one form of basic release). However, if the path keeps returning to where it came from or repeats a static cycle, the therapist can gently convert (in successive rounds) the path most insisted upon by the tissue to one of release from this trajectory.

Variations of the process can be adapted to almost any region of the anatomy because the cranial pulse radiates from the core to the limbs in its rotatory, opening-and-closing hydraulic orbit.

Craniosacral methods form a larger coherent healing system with the techniques of visceral manipulation insofar as both therapies involve palpating lines of restricted motion, inducing a response through light touch, and following tissue where it wants to go, thereby stimulating a release.

Warps, tension patterns, and pathological obstructions are all transmitted via the fascia. Fascial immobility is a guide to the exact location of disease processes hindering mobility (either at the point of stricture or elsewhere). Like the fairytale princess sensing a tiny pea under her stack of mattresses, a skilled cranial therapist can palpate through the complexity of the fascial system to the source of its distortions and immobilities, literally reaching any site in the body.

He or she will be aided by the craniosacral rhythm, both in navigating fascial pathways and in locating obstructed sites, for the fascial system complies in both gross and subtle ways with the flexion and extension of the cerebrospinal pulse.

Pulling on fascia is like stretching and twisting a bedsheet to find where it is snagged and get it free; it can be a simultaneous and complementary process to stack tissue to reach and recalibrate viscera and also to ride the hydraulics of the cranial pulse through cycles of flexion and extension. Successful palpation harmonizes elements of all these techniques in a single, highly sensitive but secure sequence of manual investigation and rebalancing.

As tensegrities of connective tissue are downplucked into microtubules, microfilaments, and the organellar anatomy of cell space, a signal starting at skin and subcutaneous muscle and nerves can distribute its kineses right into the nucleoplasm. Space and mass are arranged in perfect geometric counterpoint throughout the tissue; protein is packed in deep fractals and gapped by the infinitesimal intervals among them. Filaments and tensegrity forces open even tinier ratios within membranous stuff. The system is such a perfect resonating chamber that harmonious notes jump scale both ways and locate themselves wherever they "sound" best.

Craniosacral Therapy and Somatoemotional Release

Since the late 1980s neuropsychiatric techniques prioritizing cognitive insight, hormones, brain chemistry and the central nervous system have merged with both Eastern and Western somatic methods that empha-size the autonomic nervous system, visceral motility, and the hydro-dynamics of bodily fluids. Therapists thereby combine psychosomatic rhythms with skeletal, muscular, emotional, and spiritual aspects of tissue.

The bones, membranes, myofascia, blood-based fluids, and nerv-ous system interact to form a coherent, intelligent, self-correcting cere-brospinal network that underlies all of psychic and somatic life. Through layers of this network, the neuroses and traumas defined by psycho-therapists can also be addressed and treated.

Whereas the early osteopaths and chiropractors primarily made adjustments of skeletal-neural structures and constrictions of viscera, Upledger and his colleagues attempted to tap into the unconscious eti-ology of the whole psychosomatic field, addressing the "inner physi-cian" and encouraging it to resume or extend its native healing functions.

Insofar as the craniosacral system includes at its core the brain, spinal cord, and pituitary and pineal glands (hence the neuroendocrine system and its hormones as well as corresponding functions of the mind-body interface), it is highly sensitive to emotional components. The goal of the therapist is to find an access into psychosomatic home-ostases through palpation and to locate zones of dysfunction and restricted function within them.

Practitioners attempt to follow the myofascial, cerebrospinal web to precise historic precincts of cathected moments—or functional repli-cas of such locales—at which a malady was internalized and locked in place, sometimes embryogenically, sometimes by birth trauma, and sometimes by bodily and emotional events not fully processed. This "energy cyst" (as the somatic component of the cathexis was chris-tened by Upledger) is a multilayered knot of trapped physical and psy-chospiritual energy, functioning at a visceral and neuromuscular level, transmitting its restrictive effects fascially throughout the body (much in the way a snag at one spot in a sheet affects the contour of the entire sheet according to the intensity and direction of the snag and the texture of the material).

According to Upledger, "the complications of the Energy Cyst retention depend upon its emotional content, the quantity of energy within the cyst and its location. It seems that the emotional content of an Energy Cyst is capable of entraining the general emotional tone of the whole person. . . ."[10]

The presumption is that at an instant of traumatization, a negative energy matrix was injected into the patient's system and somaticized—the stronger the force or deeper the trauma, the more extensive and intransigent the "energy cyst" (in Upledger's terminology). The person holds onto the site emotionally through fear and anxiety, guilt, shame, grief, and even mourning and loyalty. In principle, it doesn't matter if the originating force was a gunshot wound from a carjacker, the collective deposits of years of junk food, or the humiliating taunts of a narcissistic parent. The psychophysiological environment continuously transmits immobilizing pathologies on both emotional and somatic levels through tissue and mind holistically.

One of Upledger's earliest insights is that surgeons transfer their attitudes directly through their scalpels into the tissue layers of their patients. Electrically measurable energies are transmitted directly from a physician to a patient—through hands, surgical and dental tools, and attitudes—and these energies affect healing and pathology in an explicit, quantifiable way.

Anger and disdain and, conversely, their generosity and caring are imbedded and codified in visceral memory patterns. Even the tone of a surgeon's voice while speaking idly to his assistants lodges in an anesthetized patient's tissues. Upledger found that patients could recount tales of surgical encounters with extraordinary accuracy even though they were unconscious at the time. More significantly, their bodies had somaticized the emotional tenor of the experience. "If molecularly simple recording tape has such a memory," he asks, "why not cells?"[11]

These deceptively extraneous factors determine not only the speed with which surgical wounds heal but the success of the very surgery.

When a trauma is kept from releasing, the body has to continue to function around its area of entropy. It takes energy to wall off and contain a trauma and also energy to continue to function in its context. The organism twists, oscillates, displaces itself regionally to one side or another, and hammers those twists, oscillations, and sidebends inward through tissue density. Tissue structures try to protect themselves and become knotted. Not only that, but in the formation of a wound or distortion, the body is responding instantaneously to an external force while itself moving viscerally and internally, deflecting the vectors of entry so that a linear blow from an assailant, vehicle, or stationary object bumped into imbeds itself in the system at many different angles over even milliseconds of time, much like a barbed hook fashioned to catch and hold a fish. Emotional traumas have even more complex hooks of entry through the neuromusculature.

The therapist, by tracking and unwinding somatic vectors as they lead him to their source, ultimately enters the afflicted site and then can direct his or her palpations into it at matching angles. Many ailments have multiple causes and form in layers, thus must be located in layers and cured layer by layer—the tractions always joining at the point where the various energetic sources of the condition itself meet.

If the therapist is skilled enough to track the rhythm and fascial network to traumatized sites ("energy cysts"), then the physical forces stored at those sites may be, one by one, released. The therapist does not release such energy in a predetermined fashion; instead the patient unwinds herself in response to a sympathetic palpation that guides her to her own native rhythm and movement as it responds to the healing intention behind the touch.

Energy cysts and somatoemotional traumas represent different levels of the same phenomena. The Upledger system distinguishes between a mechanical process of therapeutically releasing cysts and a more extensive procedure of full somatoemotional, post-traumatic release. The somatic component remains upstream to the emotional one, distinguishing this method from the more cognitive psychosomatic treatments of psychotherapists.

Cysts are treated first by arcing to their source (a process which in itself stimulates energetic dispersal) and then dissolving them, usually through indirect osteopathic techniques. Sometimes just holding and supporting the body at the correct point and angle (and then at each successively revealed point and angle) is sufficient to allow the viscera to release themselves. One Vietnam veteran concluded, "You can physically feel these energy cysts and physical events that have lodged themselves in you. You can literally feel them leaving your body."[12] Pieces of war that got frozen in tissue are melted and discharged. The organism knows what it needs and will often not only lead the therapist to appropriate sites but cue him in techniques by seeming to pull his hands in like suction or a magnet.

Following sensation is the key to treatment. One must avoid any prejudgment about what is functionally required for cure. In fact, techniques that shoot straight to the core may be regarded as more invasive by the patient's system and sometimes stimulate deepening of the cyst. "Don't make the patient have to defend against you," Upledger warns, "which is not the problem he came in with."[13] If the therapist makes himself the problem through overzealous "fixing" and unconscious projections, then instead of release, a new layer is added to the pathology.

Full somatoemotional cure combines physical, verbal, and emotional elements. The therapist not only diagnoses and releases cysts but guides the patient with questions about images and feelings and then, as they are answered either verbally or somatically or (usually) both, follows the new movements generated by the body wherever they go (even to entirely different energy complexes). All the time, the therapist is supporting somatic and verbal expression, following patterns, and interpolating the craniosacral rhythm as a guide.

As the craniosacral therapist steers more deeply into blocks, the patient responds by transferring the increased motility deeper. Just having his or her rhythm located and touched imparts a curative momentum both emotionally and physically in a person. The trances that arise from supporting, following, and restricting cerebrospinal flow are apparently states of grace during which unconscious communications take place and a person rearranges her entire inner being, resolving physical illnesses and traumas.

The innermost tissue layers and zones are least familiar and quite profound in terms of what they contain and can release. For the deepest reaches of the body, it is like "being seen" for the first time. After all the years of functioning in not only darkness but nullity, suddenly these texture-rich movement patterns connect to the conscious mind, the numinous "self." At the moment of becoming conscious, they "exist." As they exist, they communicate how dense and vast they actually are. Their sensations are not just the momentary static of internal exercises; they arise from the cellular basis of existence. As they differentiate from the background, they envelop the person in an awareness of whom he or she actually is and gravitate toward whom he or she might be. They literally change identity.

Whereas artificial stoppages of the craniosacral rhythm may be imposed therapeutically, the abrupt cessation of the craniosacral rhythm while "following" tissue patterns is always regarded as a deepening. Because the craniosacral system is a core system, it pulls the physician and patient inevitably to the right place (often marked by such a halt in the rhythm). At these junctures, the system simply does not know where to go. It puts out confusion. The therapist supports this place with his vector of palpation and waits for a change. Responsiveness here, remember, does not require cognitive knowledge of the cause of the trauma; palpation innately provides the visceral organization a protected way to reorder itself.

If the patient is verbally responsive at the time, the rhythm can be consulted, almost like a lie detector, to determine its truth. A full stoppage usually means "Yes!" If the patient is simultaneously experiencing an image or feeling during cessation, these are considered authentic reenactments of a traumatic source. Even if a reported image seems irrelevant at that moment to the therapist and patient, they must ignore their prejudice and trust the system. Whenever it says, "Stop here and wait," the therapist must hang out.

Though one may guess at the biological or psychospiritual agency, the fact is that the craniosacral pulse and its visceral adjuncts are branches of a pathway to the core, to a first principle of life, to the liquid light of the body-mind archetype, to its holographic patterning energies and the basis of the causal, existential realm itself. We evolved that way, and we form that way anew each time in an embryo. Without necessarily any specific hand-to-pathology blueprint, the craniosacral rhythm unwinds deeper and deeper in the sense that it contacts more and more basic coherences within the organism and ultimately transmits resolutions to stressed and dysfunctional tissue. A dialogue with the craniosacral rhythm, conducted physically, psychically, and psychologically, is a dialogue with the deepest accessible levels of an organism's existence.

Tracking another person's cranial rhythms and visceral motilities is conducting psychoanalysis nonverbally. Craniosacral therapy is like psychoanalysis in its induction of an ongoing, deepening dialogue between doctor and patient. What is astonishing is that the ostensibly mute act of osteopathic "following" replicates, as it were, psychotherapeutic discourse and transference at the level of membranes and viscera. The mere engagement of the therapist with an autonomic and seemingly unemotional rhythm appears to awaken the somatic underpinnings where emotions lodge in traumas. Guided palpation speaks to traumas in the language of their fixations and engages them along their quanta of psychosomatic potentiation. Whereas once a louder voice (letting out "the primal scream," pounding a bed with a tennis racquet, etc.) was deemed requisite to stir the demons below, now a soft touch is preferred for inducing and placating those same demons.

Craniosacral Therapy as New Science

John Upledger perceives something so obvious it is astonishing that everyone else misses it. Everyone is looking at the same thing, and some healers, physicists, and parapsychologists almost get it. Now it is gradually becoming obvious to everyone.

What Upledger sees is a world in which myriad physical, emotional, cognitive, and transpersonal factors converge to create the phenomenological human sphere. These factors are rarely considered in terms of one another, at least not in a serious medical context. They include—and I want to be careful here not to simplify Dr. Upledger's position or make him seem credulous—psychic energies, subliminal and nonconscious messages, and disembodied intelligences. Upledger has explored acupuncture, the chakra system, Kirlian photography, pyramid power, and channeled spirits. At no point, however, does he make paraphysical or hyperdimensional claims per se; he takes the spoken (and unspoken) transmissions of the human organism on their own terms—in precisely the terms they present themselves—and follows their intrinsic wisdom. He presumes that an organism's actual signs and voices are more completely organized and deeply imbedded in the ancient network we call life than any imposed external interpretations based on mechanical and purely thermodynamic views of life—or medicine.

Dr. Upledger does something so explicit and artless that it could be overlooked and yet so radical that it lies outside any contemporary paradigm—he listens to cells and tissues and tries to respond appropriately. His listening is informed medically, psychospiritually, and shamanically. He is willing to set aside his skepticism and any preexisting belief system and respond to what is happening with the person he is healing. He does not engage in speculation or medical mythodrama. He is very "nuts and bolts." The organism tells him what's going on, and he responds as best he can. Trying out the plain and self-evident and following it non-prejudicially to its natural conclusion is, sadly, rare in the world of medicine.

Here science meets religion, foreshadowing that in a true utopia or on some other world, science *is* religion. Without abandoning the skeleton and mechanical physics of tissues, osteopaths encountered a vibrating grid of life permeating everywhere—Fourth and Fifth Laws transcending ordinary thermodynamics. Still's pulleys and levers have transmuted as if through a black hole into a holistic psychotherapy as seminal as Freud's dreamwork.

In a future age, some version of craniosacral therapy may lead to the much-sought transmutative, alchemical, telekinetic science, bridging the imaginary gap between mind and body, energy and matter. That such a discovery will hearken back to the oldest Stone Age modes of touch, manipulation, voodoo, and totemic conversion will be entirely appropriate. Post-materialistic magic may regain the vitality of prescientific magic, with the additional cogency of having passed through the heart of matter, the atomic nucleus—the very birth and death of the universe—and come out the other side.

Notes

1. A. T. Still, *Osteopathy: Research & Practice* (Seattle: Eastland Press, 1992) (originally published in 1910), p. xxii.
2. Ibid., p. 19.
3. Ibid., pp. 23–24.
4. Ibid., p. xvi (foreword by Harold Goodman).
5. Hugh Milne, *The Heart of Listening: A Visionary Approach to Craniosacral Work* (Berkeley, California: North Atlantic Books, 1995), p. 55. (This and the following reference were taken from unpublished manuscript and differ slightly from the text that was later published.)
6. Ibid.
7. Rachel E. Brooks, M.D. (editor), *The Stillness of Life: The Osteopathic Philosophy of Rollin E. Becker, D.O.* (Portland, Oregon: Stillness Press, 2000), p. 178.
8. John E. Upledger, *Your Inner Physician and You: CranioSacral Therapy and SomatoEmotional Release* (Berkeley: North Atlantic Books and UI Enterprises, 1991), p. 18.
9. John E. Upledger and Jon D. Vredevoogd, *Craniosacral Therapy* (Seattle: Eastland Press, 1983), p. 9.
10. John E. Upledger, *SomatoEmotional Release and Beyond*, p. 25.
11. John Upledger, verbal communication, seminar, San Francisco, January 1994.
12. Post-Traumatic Stress Disorder in Vietnam Veterans: An Intensive CranioSacral Therapy Treatment Program.
13. John Upledger, verbal communication, seminar, San Francisco, January 1994.

Craniosacral Therapy

HANDS-ON HEALING: MASSAGE REMEDIES FOR HUNDREDS OF HEALTH PROBLEMS

You may not know it, but your head is expanding right now. In another few seconds it will start shrinking. If it's already shrinking, then it will start expanding again in just a moment.

You won't see such change in the mirror, and chances are good you could go the rest of your life without noticing it and never lose a good night's sleep. Maybe.

But, if you've ever suffered from such things as migraine headaches, temporomandibular joint (TMJ) dysfunction, ringing in the ears, dyslexia, depression, or any number of chronic aches and pains throughout your body, then the fact that your head expands and contracts at a rate of 8 to 12 times a minute could become quite important to you.

In fact, this knowledge, combined with the skilled touch of someone practicing a hands-on healing technique known as craniosacral therapy, might help provide relief from many such disorders. And that could be worth a good night's sleep.

Cranial Respiration

Craniosacral therapists lightly work with the bones of the skull. In so doing they also work with the membranes beneath the skull that sup-

Reprinted with permission from John Feltman, ed., *Hands-On Healing: Massage Remedies for Hundreds of Health Problems* (Emmaus, PA: Rodale Press, 1989), 66–74.

port the brain, as well as the cerebrospinal fluid that cushions and bathes the brain and spinal cord from cranium to sacrum.

In much the same way that contracting your calf muscles helps move blood in the lower legs back to the heart, craniosacral therapists believe that the motion of the skull helps move cerebrospinal fluid around your brain and down your spine to the sacrum, which gently rocks in rhythm with the motions of the skull.

But these therapists also believe that all the bumps, bruises, and sharp blows to the head you've received since the day you were born have probably knocked some of those bones out of alignment, causing them to freeze up or move improperly.

By gently manipulating the skull bones at the sutures (those fibrous joints that hold bones together in the skull), craniosacral therapists seek to realign the bones so that they move in sync with one another, allowing the cerebrospinal fluid to circulate freely. During the manipulation process, therapists also remove the stresses that accumulate in the membranes supporting and surrounding the brain and spinal column.

As Jim Asher, of the Colorado Cranial Institute in Boulder, explains: "We're moving fluid, rebalancing fluid, stretching membranes, and sometimes balancing bones."

Exactly why this stretching and balancing produces the results it does is still a matter of some speculation. "I can't answer questions with the word 'exactly' in them," says John Upledger, DO, a craniosacral instructor and director of The Upledger Institute in Palm Beach Gardens, Florida.

"In some cases manipulation might increase the circulation of the cerebrospinal fluid," he says, "but the primary goal is to mobilize the system. What we want is to see that system moving symmetrically and without a lot of resistance to its activity. The benefit of that can be as far reaching as taking away a chronic pain in your left leg."

Meant for Motion

Though craniosacral therapy started out as a branch of osteopathy, the inability of its practitioners to explain exactly how the technique works hurt its popularity. But even more than the mysterious nature of its healing powers, there's another, more basic reason why you've probably never heard of craniosacral therapy before.

As noted above, craniosacral therapists believe the bones in your skull were meant for motion, and they use their gentle, hands-on technique to help increase and synchronize that motion. But Gray's Anatomy (the bible of anatomical reference books), along with most other anatomy texts, says the bones of the skull are immobile. Many doctors agree, implying that any therapy based on movable skull bones must clearly be nonsense.

But the massage therapists, osteopathic physicians, and physicians who do practice craniosacral therapy disagree with the accepted view of cranial immobility. They point instead to the teachings of William G. Sutherland, a turn-of-the-century osteopathic physician whose ideas about flexible sutures and cranial movement have only recently been subjected to serious, scientific scrutiny.

Dr. Sutherland believed that the skull moved in response to the body's production of cerebrospinal fluid deep inside the ventricles of the brain. He theorized that the ventricles pulse as they release cerebrospinal fluid, increasing the hydraulic pressure inside the skull and causing it to expand.

Dr. Sutherland wondered what would happen if the skull bones were prevented from moving, and wrapped his head with bandages in order to find out. The result was "an immediate change of the movement of the diaphragmatic respiratory mechanism," he wrote. This sudden change that Dr. Sutherland noted in his breathing pattern helped convince him that the cranial respiratory system was "the primary respiratory mechanism" of the body, and that breathing was, in his words, "secondary thereto."

The idea that the skull was designed to expand and contract and that the craniosacral system was the primary respiratory system of the body did little to endear Dr. Sutherland to mainstream medical practitioners.

He did, however, obtain some fairly remarkable results with his cranial work, and detailed the technique in a small book called *The Cranial Bowl,* which he filled with case histories. Recently, an interdisciplinary team of osteopathic physicians, anatomists, biophysicists, and others at the Department of Biomechanics at Michigan State University's College of Osteopathic Medicine launched a scientific investigation of Dr. Sutherland's work, determined to put his theories to the test once and for all.

Dr. Upledger was a member of the Michigan State investigating team. "The department said we're either going to prove it true or prove it false," he says, "so we started looking." The result: "We found that it had a pretty good scientific base."

An Uphill Battle

Indeed, just about everyone who has seriously examined Dr. Sutherland's theories has concluded that he was correct, and that restrictions in the craniosacral rhythm may be implicated in such things as migraines, depression, cerebral palsy, and more.

Does that mean you'll be able to walk into an osteopathic physician's office and request a session of craniosacral therapy? Hardly.

Notes Stephen Blood, DO, president of the Cranial Academy in Meridian, Idaho, an organization dedicated to furthering the cause of craniosacral therapy among osteopathic physicians: "It is still practiced in our profession, but it is practiced by a small minority of the 24,000 osteopathic physicians in the country."

Small minority is right. The Cranial Academy has fewer than 300 members. And, as Dr. Blood points out, it wages an uphill battle in trying to popularize the technique with the many osteopathic physicians who've never tried craniosacral therapy.

"For one, it takes a level of palpatory skill that's not there for everyone," he explains. "Also, it's very time consuming and it's not cost-effective for the osteopathic physician. You could normally see two or three patients in the time that it takes to do a single session of cranial work."

Dr. Upledger agrees. "I book patients at 45-minute intervals when I'm doing cranial work. Most osteopathic physicians aren't going to spend 45 minutes with a patient."

As a result, craniosacral work is now practiced mostly by physical therapists, massage professionals, and other bodywork specialists, many of whom routinely spend an hour or more with individual clients and think nothing of it.

Many of Asher's students at the Colorado Cranial Institute are massage professionals who have experienced craniosacral therapy as clients and simply want to add it to their repertoire. "Basically," Asher explains, "the students come in and study for about four days, then they go out and practice for three to six months."

Students eventually progress from the basic level to intermediate and advanced. The total time involved can vary from a year to 18 months, depending on the student's progress and the amount of time spent in practice between levels. The school has been in existence since 1980.

Dr. Upledger's school utilizes the same basic format as Asher's, with some minor variations. "We have four levels," he says. "People take an introductory seminar, then go out and practice a few months. They come back and we give them an intermediate seminar. They practice that, and then there are two more levels they go through. It's about 20 days of training over a year or year and a half."

Dr. Upledger says his students are primarily physical therapists, chiropractors, MDs, or DOs. The Upledger Institute has been in existence for about four years, and Upledger estimates that more than 2,000 people have attended his training seminars to date.

Both Dr. Upledger and Asher agree that the most important skill any craniosacral student can possess, regardless of background, is "very good palpatory ability, or the ability to develop it."

A Keen Sense of Touch

Dan Matarazzo has been practicing craniosacral therapy for the past four years in Tucson, Arizona. He developed his "palpatory ability" at the Colorado Cranial Institute, and like many of its graduates, he mixes cranial work with other techniques. In Matarazzo's case it's Rolfing, a deep tissue technique that, while effective, can be uncomfortable for some people.

Matarazzo says that craniosacral therapy can be a very beneficial technique for patients who suffer from shyness and who are unable to relax in typical massage settings.

"Cranial work can be done on people who are fully clothed," he explains. "On the other hand, something like Rolfing is a much more direct intervention in the body and it's usually done in your underwear. There are some people who are just not ready for that. So, where it's applicable, I use cranial work instead and find it really effective."

One of craniosacral therapy's most effective applications, Matarazzo says, is with TMJ-related jaw pain: "I see a lot of occipital and temporal problems, with the temporals leading to TMJ problems." (The temporal bones are located on the side of the skull, around the ears.

The occipital bone is located in the lower back part of the skull, where it wraps around to join the temporals.)

Like most craniosacral practitioners, Matarazzo uses his keen sense of touch to detect problems throughout the body, even though his hands never leave the skull. "I see a lot of people with occipital problems that tell me they have some pelvic problems as well. There's a real relationship between the occiput and the sacrum. You can tell what's going on in the pelvis by the way the occiput is sitting."

Not surprising, perhaps, Matarazzo finds headaches the easiest malady for cranial work to treat. "The hardest things tend to be old head injuries that the patient may have internalized and may not even be aware of," he says.

Like Matarazzo, Theresa Pearce is trained in both craniosacral therapy and Rolfing. Unlike Matarazzo, however, this Grand Rapids, Michigan, practitioner never combines the two therapies for use on the same patient.

"Most of those who come to me for cranial work come because of stress, chronic headaches, or neck pain," she says. "They are the type of people who can't seem to let go and relax."

Pearce also finds that craniosacral therapy is effective on TMJ pain. She believes most TMJ problems can be traced back to birth trauma. "I'm 33, and a lot of people from my generation have gone through forceps deliveries," she says. "You can see that in people, the way their skulls are pressed in on the sides, and the way a lot of them have TMJ symptoms now."

Craniosacral and Kids

The trauma placed on the human skull during birth has been a subject of natural fascination for craniosacral therapists. One of the first osteopathic physicians to explore and apply cranial work to young children was Dr. Beryl F. Arbuckle, a pediatrician who studied with Dr. Sutherland and soon became one of craniosacral therapy's most vocal proponents.

Dr. Arbuckle applied Dr. Sutherland's techniques to the management of cerebral palsy cases, and with great success. As her fame grew, she began treating patients from all over the world and was eventually awarded osteopathic medicine's highest honor, the Andrew Taylor Still Medallion. Even so, her method of treatment—craniosacral therapy—languished in obscurity.

The use of this technique for treating children has not been completely forgotten or abandoned, however. "Cranial manipulation and pediatrics just go hand-in-hand," says the Cranial Academy's Dr. Blood. "I can't imagine being able to work on children and not taking advantage of it."

And neither, it seems, can pediatrician Paul Dunn, one of the few MDs in the nation who uses craniosacral therapy in his practice. "The first time I heard of it was in 1969," recalls the Oak Park, Illinois, physician. "A family came in with a severely brain damaged child and said that an osteopathic physician was manipulating the child's skull bones. They asked me what I thought of it. I told them I really didn't think it could be done, but if they thought it was helping, go ahead."

Several years later, in 1974, Dr. Dunn attended a medical meeting where he met an osteopathic physician who was using the technique in his practice. His interest was piqued. After visiting extensively with one of the osteopathic physicians, Dr. Dunn decided to learn the technique himself. "It's been 14 years now and I'm quite pleased with it," he says.

Dr. Dunn incorporates craniosacral work into the holistic approach he takes when treating children. "We use it as part of the picture," he explains. "But the kids we use it on are those who have brain injuries, developmental delays, hyperactivity, and so on. In itself it is not a cure-all, but it is a very useful adjunct to the other types of treatment we do."

For the last eight years, Dr. Dunn has also been using craniosacral therapy as part of his approach to help adult patients suffering from long-standing fatigue, depression, headaches, gastrointestinal problems, and other problems.

Craniosacral Resources

For more information on craniosacral therapy:

COLORADO CRANIAL INSTITUTE
466 Marine Street
Boulder, CO 80302
(303) 447-2760

EXECUTIVE DIRECTOR
The Cranial Academy
1140 West Eighth Street
Meridian, ID 83642
(208) 888-1201

THE UPLEDGER INSTITUTE
11211 Prosperity Farms Road
Palm Beach Gardens, FL 33410
(407) 622-4334

The following books can provide additional background:

The Cranial Bowl by William G. Sutherland
(Free Press Co.)

Craniosacral Therapy by John Upledger
and Jon Vredevoogd (Eastland)

Despite such stories of positive results, there's little chance of craniosacral therapy gaining widespread popularity in the medical community any time soon.

Dr. Dunn estimates that the number of MDs who use craniosacral therapy "are relatively few."

The Healing Power of Craniosacral Therapy

The lights are dim, the padded bench soft. You close your eyes as the craniosacral therapist seated behind you grasps your head and begins manipulating the eight bones of your skull. The grip, strengthened by years of practice, is firm, but the touch is incredibly light.

"This can't possibly be doing anything," you think to yourself. A minute later you hear yourself snoring and realize that somehow, somewhere, some part of you is asleep. That realization makes whatever part of your brain that was dozing snap back to consciousness.

The hands have moved from the back of your skull to the sides, pulling at the large parietal bones near the top of your head. You feel completely calm and serene, though you realize you only met the person tugging on your head an hour ago. By the time that thought starts to sink in you're sleeping again, one part of your brain snoring away while the other part listens and feels almost embarrassed, never having heard itself snore before.

The rest of the session is more of the same. Lapses of consciousness followed by dreams.

"It was like I was there but I wasn't there," recalls Margaret Long, a Grand Rapids patient of Theresa Pearce. "It was almost as though I had been drugged. I was aware of what was going on in the room, but I wasn't there.

"I must sound like some kind of space cadet," Long laughs. "I'm the type of person who always has to be in control, but going through something like that was really nice for me."

Also nice was the way craniosacral therapy relieved Long's pain: "I have always had a lot of headaches," she says. "Whenever Theresa's done work on me, it's always been for neck or head pain and it's always been very effective. All the tension that builds up in my face and jaw and the back of my head is released, and the relief lasts about a week or so—which is pretty long-term relief when compared with taking painkillers every day."

Patricia Merkle has been visiting Dan Matarazzo for the past two years. "He alternates Rolfing and craniosacral work with me, depending on what he feels needs to be done," she says.

"It's really pleasant, really relaxing," Merkle says of the craniosacral work she has had. "Sometimes I drift off and I'm not there at all. Other times my mind sticks around and I can feel what he's doing and know what is going on." Merkle says she prefers the craniosacral work for its relaxing properties, relying on the deep tissue work of Rolfing for relief from physical maladies.

Even so, she says cranial work has also brought about some fairly surprising physical releases. "I've felt a hip release and a leg release after having the joint freeze or stiffen up," Merkle says. "It's the type of thing you might treat with a heating pad, but with the craniosacral work it's an instantaneous release—you don't have to wait for it to happen."

Merkle and Long both realize that relatively few others have ever experienced the subtle powers of this gentle healing art. "Cranial work comes to people when they are ready for it," says Long. "If someone came to me and said he had some headaches, I might try to explain craniosacral to him, but if I got a puzzled look or any negative feedback, I'd just stop talking about it." Unfortunately, that seems to be the way it's gone with craniosacral therapy all along.

Hands-On Techniques

The following illustrations depict procedures used by trained craniosacral therapists. They are not intended for do-it-yourself applications.

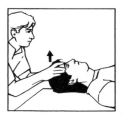

Figure 10-1 The craniosacral therapist places his hands near the temples and lifts upward, decompressing the frontal bone and stretching the membrane beneath. This move, a frontal lift, is used to help relieve eye strain and sinus pressure.

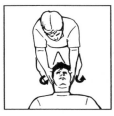

Figure 10-2 Here, the therapist places his hands on the temporal bones and, through manipulation, helps bring them back into balance. This move is used to help alleviate ringing in the ears.

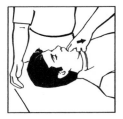

Figure 10-3 This rather bizarre-looking technique, in which the jawbone is stretched to its limit, is used for relieving temporomandibular joint (TMJ) pain.

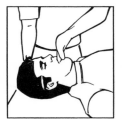

Figure 10-4 The therapist applies pressure to the bones in the roof of the mouth, balancing the upper jaw and bringing relief to the maxillary sinuses.

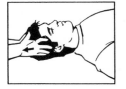

Figure 10-5 The parietal lift helps balance the large parietal bones on either side of the skull and stretches the membrane beneath, to help relieve headache pain and stress.

Philosophies, Stories, and Lessons

JOHN E. UPLEDGER

CranioSacral therapy has been my life's work, and I've come to realize that it arises from openness. The whole thing in a nutshell, doing this work, is you put your hands on and you blend. You be one with the person you're working on. The intelligence of that person starts coming through into you and it comes into your consciousness. Then if you're smart enough not to follow your rationality, you just do it.

I don't have preconceived notions. When a person lies on the table, I don't want to know what's the matter. I want to evaluate him or her first and then we go from there. I'm just doing what I'm told. The patient's body is where the information comes from.

The refusal to admit, let alone explore, this is just about the biggest problem I have with conventional medicine. Arrogance has to be totally dismissed. You have to let go of your ego completely and you have to be like a blank check that can be used in a lot of ways. It's acceptable here, here, here—but it's always blank. She's going to put the writing on it. That's how it works.

I'll give for an example of a brand new patient I've had. The diagnosis she brought with her is pseudotumor of the spinal cord. Pseudo is fake; what it means is that there's fluid involved in a cystic apparatus, but there's no cell or tissue in there to make it a tumor. It's just fluid. They call it a pseudotumor. Back when I was working at Sun Coast Hospital in Clearwater, Florida, I used to operate with the neurosurgeon, and we did some pseudotumors. In those days, you used x-ray because that's the only thing you had. The pseudotumor looked like a tumor because the dye that you used in the x-ray went around it. The assumption was that it was a tumor, but invariably it was a cyst. They called it a pseudotumor because it's, in a way, an imitation of tumor. I've seen enough of them that when I hear a diagnosis of pseudotumor, what that means to me is that they don't know what it is, but it looks like it's got fluid in it.

With this woman, it was pretty easy. She had tremendous pain from this place, coming around from the front of her chest, and it was about the level of sixth to the eleventh thoracic. It was on the righthand side and it was about an inch wide. I picked this up from my own feelings about what I was contacting. As I got the fluid out of there. she began feeling better immediately. I've worked on her three or four times now. We just treated it like a cystic tumor that's full of cerebrospinal fluid rather than tissue. We get that to move out and stay out. The whole point is, if I can flatten it and then hold it flattened for a while, it will begin to glue itself together and not be pushed apart by the fluid pressure.

When I treat her, I put a hand in the back and a hand in the front and I imagine energy going through there that will move the fluid. This is what I'm talking about when I describe passing energy in CST. Let me explain it in another way. I've been reading about quantum physics, and I'm a big fan of Erwin Schrödinger. In the early 1900s he wrote the first formula to be accepted in quantum physics. He got a Nobel Laureate for it. What I'm coming up with very much resembles his model of waves, particles, and uncertainty theory; that is, if I want something to disappear, I put enough energy through it, and what happens is, astonishingly, it disappears. That how strong intention is—it works on a quantum level.

Anything that is clogging a system—even fluid—is of course made up of atoms. Every electron in an atom has a specific electrical charge, and it's always negative. The neutron and the proton in the nucleus of the atom are made up of quarks; each quark has exactly the same positive charge as the electron has a negative one. What happens when I put a lot of energy through living matter in the form of intention is that the energy increases the activity of the atoms and of the quantum quarks. When an electron and a quark collide they lose their mass and turn into energy. Now what I'm doing is sending quanta of subtle heat energy that increase the amount of this activity. That means there are more collisions between positive and negative particles and anti-particles and, when they collide, they turn into energy and lose their mass. The energy comes out as heat. When you're doing this and you're feeling the heat coming out, you're engaged in a quantum process.

Entropy is the negative energy that causes things to age, to ultimately die or fall apart. It's countered by what Schrödinger called information, aka syntropy, which is the part that keeps you alive. The balance between entropy and syntropy is going to dictate whether you're going to be degrading or revitalizing. Schrödinger also said that when you feel the heat come out, it's bringing entropy with it and therefore you're revitalizing wherever it came from.

Between those two concepts—the heat coming out and the quarks and electrons turning into energy and then removing entropy—probably there is some unknown connection. The entropy and the quark electron activity are related. I'm willing to guess that they are probably different ways of looking at the same central phenomenon but coming in from two divergent directions. Anyway that's what I'm doing with this patient. I'm dissolving the fluid in her pseudotumor and, at the same time, I'm trying to get rid of the entropy that prevents the tissue from healing back together again.

It's all my intention. That's it. That's as far as I can go—and I really don't give a damn whether the quantum stuff or any other story about why something happens is true or not. If I intend it and it works, I don't need to know more than that. If I am blessed and I wake up one morning after a dream about something and understand how to do it, that's wonderful. We are not automatons; we are mysterious beings with many dimensions. I don't need a statistical survey or lab test to tell me what I know or what I don't know or what I supposedly can't know. Dreams, intuitions, and listening are the way I get most of my information. Sometimes I just awake in the morning with it. You put your intention where you want it.

Does that ever piss scientists off! They're still trying to do a double-blind study, double-blind on the universe—but it's impossible. They find out that one guy feels palpation and the other guy feels something else, so it must be nothing.

My point is, I'm using my intuition to get into the fluid and to dissolve it and get it to turn into energy, using the principles that I just gave you. Physicists don't get challenged on hypotheses like relativity or quantum theory or uncertainty principle, but if you put something like that out in medicine, they'll crucify you. Whether these things are true or not, they heal people. That's what counts for me. I don't need to be able to go all the way with it. There are too many sick people needing our help to waste time with academic experiments. We're doctors, not accountants.

A lot of my ideas go all the way back to Dr. Howell at Kirksville. He taught me about scale; everything recapitulates itself at different intervals of scale. The atom has a nucleus. If you look at it in a bigger arena, the nucleus is the sun and the electrons are the planets. If you want to understand life, Dr. Howell taught me, you have to understand size and domain.

Usually my general methods tend not to make scientists happy, but then again, more and more as the years go by, that's improved, and the world has begun to change. We've had a few neurosurgeons taking our curriculum. We get more cooperation from them than some specialists; generally, neurosurgeons don't feel as though we're getting on their turf. A neurosurgeon will do surgery and then sometimes send his patient down here for CranioSacral work because that will help the surgery, and it makes him look good too. But, at the same time, he doesn't want to know what we're really doing.

I shouldn't generalize. We've had just three neurosurgeons who have taken our classes and they're fine with this stuff. The neurologists are the ones who really hate me. They hoard their incurable diseases. They'll tell you this is terminal, this is irreversible, and then their patients come down here in panic and we reverse the damned things. Boy, that really honks them off. I've had neurologists call me and put me through quizzes about, do you know where this nerve goes, do you know what that nerve does, do you know where the nerve centers are, etc.? I'll say, "Is this a State board to renew my license or something?" I get smart with them. I haven't met a conventional physician yet who scared me.

The Nature of Palpation

DON COHEN

Human physiology exists perpetually in the fluid state; that is, it fluxes constantly as it processes, moves, and copes. Palpation offers us a means by which we can appreciate physiology in the fluid state, a means that is "totally subjective and completely reliable" (Upledger).

Passive and Active Palpation: The Fluid Nature of Rhythm

Active palpation utilizes the application of digital pressure (pacinian corpuscles) or movement to assess parameters such as range of motion, pain sensitivity, shape, consistency, muscle tension, etc., and may induce a response or movement in the subject.

Passive palpation utilizes minimal pressure and movement so that the physiologic motion of the whole organism can be appreciated in a relatively undisturbed state. In developing appreciation of the craniosacral rhythm and other subtle motions of the organism, passive palpation is the choice. Because we are perceiving wave motion through a liquid medium it is best to avoid setting any extraneous waves into motion with our palpation. Active palpation used inappropriately may also induce a defensive tension response in the neuromusculature of the subject, and this tension will tend to interfere with the tissue's ability to transmit the inherent wave activity accurately. Lastly, motion on the part of the palpator involves motor activity of the palpating hand and competes with the perception of the sensory tracts.

Palpating the Continuum: Gross to Subtle

The body represents a spectrum of tissue density from gross to subtle. Hard tissue, soft tissue, membrane tension patterns, fluid wave patterns, and subtle energy can all be palpated. The craniosacral rhythm represents a unifying wave pattern through the spectrum of densities. The ability to grasp the continuum of this spectrum at once, as it exists, offers us the opportunity to appreciate the patient in a way not available by any other means.

TABLE I: **The Spectrum of Densities**

Gross . . . . Subtle
bone
soft tissue
membrane tension
fluid wave patterns

Note: "Energy" in humans refers to behavior (activity) and to the ability (potential) to behave. Behavior may be willful, "subconscious," or autonomic. Autonomic energy (activity) tends to move in patterns (rhythm). Organization of activity is the basis of good function, the "secret" of good health.

Proprioceptive and Tactile Palpation

There are two primary conscious sensory pathways in the CNS.

The **spinothalamic** tract transmits **exteroceptive** sensations which arise from stimuli outside the self. These include pain, temperature, and objective touch. The spinothalamic fibers cross in the cord and ascend to the thalamus. This tract is also responsible for viscerosomatic sensations and plays a role in the "gating" mechanism of pain limitation.

The **dorsal column-lemniscal** pathway carries conscious **proprioceptive** sensations which arise within the body, including sense of position of the musculoskeletal components at rest, kinesthetic sense of the body in motion, and vibratory sensation (pattern organization of touch). It also has tactile discrimination fibers which define the subjective tactile sense, including that of texture and pressure. This pathway ascends in the dorsal columns of the cord and crosses in the medulla oblongata just before synapsing at the nuclei cuneatus and gracilis. It then proceeds as the medial lemniscus to the thalamus. **Interoception** refers to the autonomic ascending pathways.

There is a third spinocerebellar pathway for unconscious proprioception, which is in intimate communication with the conscious sense. The two pathways of conscious perception provide the basis of the bipalpatory concept.

TABLE 2: **Conscious Sensory Routes**

TRACTS

Spinothalamic	Dorsal column-lemniscal
exteroception	conscious proprioception
objective touch (stereognosis)	subjective touch (and fine gradation)
pain (nociception)	body position at rest
thermal	kinesthetic sense
viscerosomatic	vibratory (pattern of pressure and touch)
poor spatial definition	spatially specific (homunculus)
slow (1–15 mps)	fast (30–75 mps)

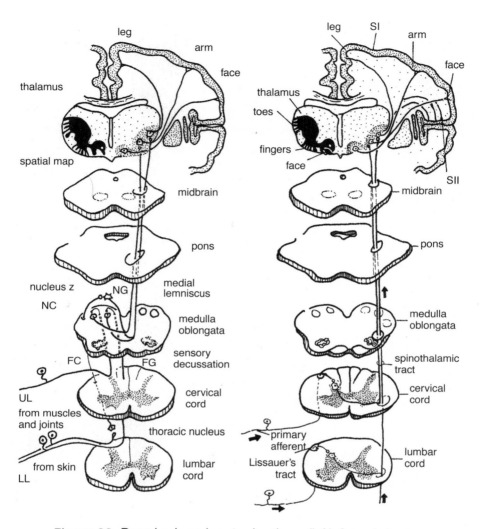

Figure 23 Dorsal column-lemniscal pathway (left). Spinothalamic tract (right)

The active palpating hand utilizes motor activity (movement and pressure) and sensory activity (tactile discrimination) to discriminate between its activity and that of the subject, as perceived at the boundary between palpator and subject. It is a probe, and its nature is to "delve into" tissue and discover information. Objective tactile discrimination is exteroceptive and occurs at the dermal and epidermal level (body surface) with the activation of tactile skin receptors.

The Vibratory Sense

The vibratory sense perceives organization in biphasic touch activity (rhythm). The rhythm can be binary (digital) or wave-form (analog) and may be easily organized or may seem random. Vibratory sensation ascends with the proprioceptive tracts.

The Blended Hand

The passive palpating hand "blends" with the subject, bypassing the tactile receptors. When learning to palpate proprioceptively, it is useful to avoid focusing on the hands at first. Use the proprioceptive mechanism of your wrists, forearms, elbows, and arms as your main sensory instrument. From this vantage the hand proprioceptors are also readily available, especially in the interossei and opponens muscles.

It is the proprioceptive tracts that allow us to know our own body position in the dark. Most of us regard this as a sensitive and absolutely reliable system. The blended hand is by its quiet nature fully sensory, and as it is also fluid it rides with the wave pattern of that with which it is blended. In proprioceptive palpation, discriminate between one part of yourself (distal forearm/wrist, elbow) and another (proximal forearm/elbow) as a means of understanding the milieu of your subject. The dorsal columns provide us with "an instantaneous body image at the level of the somatic sensory cortex" (Fitzgerald). The development of this conscious and inherent imaging phenomenon, in conjunction with the blended hand, allows us to perceive our patient in a subjective physiologic state. The human nervous system is as complex and sensitive a sensory device as has ever been devised "by God or Man." There are myriad implications to the old adage "Know yourself" in this practice.

Subjectivity in Palpation

The nervous system is a specialized communication system. Palpation is a purely subjective skill that allows us to communicate with the nervous system itself. The willfulness of the human central nervous system is well documented. As the experience of life, conscious and autonomic, is largely subjective it seems appropriate that this appreciation be developed. Passive palpation is listening and requires presence. Perhaps the less one says about what he palpates, the better we can trust that person's palpatory efficacy. The idea is not to give the patient advice, but to listen as the patient expresses herself, something she does inherently every moment of her life. In chiropractic we call this innate intelligence.

Training the Senses

For the purpose of training ourselves to utilize proprioceptive palpation, the exercises below will discourage the use of active palpation. The clinical practitioner of course takes appropriate advantage of both active and passive palpation, and with the acquisition of skill learns to appreciate both sensory tracts simultaneously with the motor function.

The Sensory Basis of Motor Function: The Long Loop

Inherent to the motor function is the concept of intent. Intentional use of the body derives neurologically from the motor cortex and beyond that from a nebulous locale, the place in us where thought originates. Afferent impulses to the motorneurons also originate from the sensory tracts as either cord reflex or **"long loop"** reflex via the dorsal column-lemniscal pathway to the sensorimotor cortex. In this way intentional motor activity relies on feedback mechanisms from that which we feel. The **long loop** pathway involves a conscious sensory tract and a conscious motor tract. (It also plays a major role in muscle testing.) Train your focus on the long loop for palpation. The implication, of course, is that in delivering care to your patient, the motor function actively relies on the proprioceptive reality of the patient's physiologic state, and this allows a more direct communication with the patient.

Selective Focus

The craniosacral, vascular, and breathing rhythms can all be palpated from any vantage. Train yourself to bring your attention to any one aspect of this phenomenon and then "wipe clean" your sentient field and refocus on another aspect. Thus from any listening station you can perceive first the vascular pulsations, then the breathing rhythm, and then the craniosacral rhythm, and switch back and forth among them at will. Selective focus also allows you to alternate between exteroceptive and proprioceptive sensory circuits as you palpate.

Palpation of Poise

Poise is the resting attitude of the organism. Poise is physical (body habitus), mental (thought), and emotional (feeling). Structural poise is the way the body holds itself at rest (in neutral), including all of the joint relationships, muscle tension patterns, etc. Poise cannot be described, predicted, or quantified. Aspects of poise can be measured but are in all cases inefficient in relating the essence of its nature. Poise can be palpated proprioceptively as a spontaneous impression. Let it in. Focusing your attention on poise enables you to "lock in" to the tension pattern of your patient so that you can interact with it.

Practice: Proprioceptive Perception

Two partners.

Partner A: Hold your hands out, palms up.

Partner B: Your hands rest on your partner's hands. Relax your hands and keep your touch light.

A: Rotate your hands gently to approximate the Cranial Respiratory Impulse. See how subtle a motion you can create.

B: Close your eyes and feel the motion in your forearms and elbows. See how subtle a motion you can perceive.

Practice: Membrane Tension

Three partners. These short and simple exercises demonstrate the straightforward concept of palpating membrane tension. It can be just about this easy to feel distal tension in the body. These same exercises are also included in the chapter on reciprocal tension.

1) A and B: Hold the corners of a sheet of plastic wrap and pull it taut. Each partner can slightly exaggerate the pull on one corner for a moment to demonstrate reciprocal tension.

C: Poke the "membrane" gently with your finger from above and below. See how subtle an interference you can create.

A and B: With your eyes closed, identify the location of the finger. See how subtle an interference you can identify.

C: Now poke your finger at an angle to introduce a vector component.

2) A and B: Same as above.

C: Hold your open hand to the surface of the membrane.

A and B: Create reciprocal tension from the corners of the membrane. Add additional vectors with a free finger while C identifies the source of the interference.

Practice: Palpation of Poise and Rhythms on Self

Sit comfortably and raise your arms. Bend your elbows and place your hands gently on your head with your fingers comfortably spread. Your wrists are suspended like slings from your elbows. With your touch as light as possible, alight on the skull like water spiders on surface tension. Your thumbs are under your occipital base and your fifth fingers grace the sides of your frontal. Rest at the interface of your scalp and the atmosphere, and then settle in to the skull. Relax and register your physical impression, the poise of the total skull. Imagine for a moment the structural architecture that you know underlies this feeling. All of the joint relationships throughout the body structure refer directly to the body poise because together they create it. The fluid and membrane of the soft tissue push and pull distinctively.

Now bring your attention to the rhythm of your breath. The breathing rhythm subtly nods the head (rocking of the occipital condyles on the superior articular facets of the atlas).

Wipe your focus clean and pick up the arterial pulsation in the scalp. It should be easy to identify. Listen to it for a while, then wipe your focus clean once again and listen for the craniosacral respiratory impulse. The CRI is palpated as a widening and shortening, then a narrowing and lengthening of the skull. It can be deduced from the pendular motion in your relaxed elbows as they rock subtly back and forth. Now feel the motion in your scapulae as they float in and out in synch with your elbows. In this way, register the craniosacral rhythm in your body. The use of your tactile proprioceptive pathway amplifies your own subjective joint proprioception. Each phase of cranial flexion or extension normally takes about three seconds. When you have registered the rhythm, feel it without judgement for a few minutes. Then begin to note the amplitude and symmetry of the impulse. Practice switching back and forth among the three rhythms at will, wiping your sentient (perceptive) field clean between perceptions.

Now return to poise without losing the rhythm. From your palpatory vantage, imagine the poise of the entire body architecture as it relates to your tactile impression. This exercise strengthens your intuition.

Practice: Cranial Rhythm on a Subject

Sit at the head of the table. Your subject is supine. Cradle your subject's head comfortably in your hands, with the ears between the third and fourth fingers (vault hold). Palpate the cranial rhythm for a minute, your blended hands doing what the head is doing. Suspend your elbows and feel the rhythm in them. Notice that you can feel a slight motion in your own arms and in your pectorals. Now "ride" with the rhythm. Get ahead of it by anticipating it just slightly as it flexes and extends, as though the hands welcome and encourage the motion. Now confront the fulcrum; anticipating the maximum motion, resist the last bit of motion not by pushing but by becoming "immoveable as stone." Confront the edge of each phase and let it push up against the "stone" of your hand. Then let it up, and "welcome" it again, riding for several cycles. Now you are ready to practice the palpation of rhythms at the various listening stations of the body. This is the preliminary skill required for working with the craniosacral system.

Craniosacral Therapy

NATIONAL INSTITUTES OF HEALTH

Craniosacral therapy is a gentle, hands-on treatment method that focuses on alleviating restrictions to physiological motion of all the bones of the skull, including the face and mouth, as well as the vertebral column, sacrum, coccyx, and pelvis. Concurrently, the craniosacral therapist focuses as well on normalizing abnormal tensions and stresses in the meningeal membrane, with special attention to the outermost membrane, the dura mater, and its fascial connections. Attention is also paid to alleviating any obstacles to free movement by the cerebrospinal fluid within its membrane compartment and to normalizing and balancing perceived related energy fields. This approach is derived from experiments of John Upledger, an osteopathic physician and researcher (for example, see Upledger, 1977a and 1977b, which are discussed below).

As usually practiced, this therapy is a noninvasive treatment process that requires an uninterrupted treatment session of at least 30 minutes; often the session is extended beyond an hour. Practitioners indicate that successful treatment relies largely on the therapist's ability to facilitate the patient's own self-corrective processes within the craniosacral system. Postgraduate training in craniosacral therapy has been undertaken by a wide variety of physicians, dentists, and therapists. In the United States during 1993, 2,738 health care professionals completed

Reprinted from National Institutes of Health, *Alternative Medicine: Expanding Medical Horizons. A Report to the National Institutes of Health on Alternative Medical Systems and Practices in the United States* (Washington, DC: U.S. Government Printing Office, 1994), NIH Publication No. 94-066, 148–149.

the Upledger Institute's introductory-level workshop and seminar; 1,827 received training at the intermediate level; and 80 completed the advanced level. Training outside this country is available through the Upledger Institute Europe in the Netherlands and on a smaller scale in Japan, New Zealand, France, and Norway by American Upledger Institute teachers.

The most powerful effects of craniosacral therapy are considered to be on the function of the central nervous system, the immune system, the endocrine system, and the visceral organs via the autonomic nervous system. This therapy has been used with reported success in many cases of brain and spinal cord dysfunction. Although these successes have not been documented in formal studies, they have been observed subjectively or anecdotally by both patients and therapists. Most prominent among these success reports are cases of brain injury resulting in symptoms of spastic paralysis and seizure. Other areas of claimed success include cerebral palsy, learning disabilities, seizure disorders, depressive reactions, menstrual dysfunction, motor dysfunction, strabismus (a vision disorder), temporomandibular joint problems, various headaches, chronic pain problems, and chronic fatigue syndrome.

Research on tissues has documented the potential for movement between skull bones in adult humans, and pilot work with live primates has shown rhythmical movement of their skull bones. Interrater reliability studies, which look for correlations in the observations of two or more independent raters . . . , have shown agreement between "blinded" therapists evaluating preschool-aged children ("blinding" means that the therapists making the observations did not know which children had received craniosacral therapy, nor did they know the history or problems of the children) (Upledger, 1977a). Controlled studies have shown high correlation between schoolchildren with various brain dysfunctions and specific dysfunctions of the craniosacral system; that is, the craniosacral exam scores correlated with recorded school teacher and psychologist opinions of "not normal," behavioral problems, motor coordination problems, learning disabilities, and obstetrical complications (Upledger, 1977b). Moreover, Upledger reports that a few pilot studies by dentists have demonstrated significant changes in the transverse dimension of the hard palate as well as in occlusion in response to craniosacral therapy.

At present, work is under way that appears to demonstrate fluctuations in what are called energy measurements in circuits between craniosacral therapists and patients. The circuits are established by attaching electrodes to the patient and the therapist with an ohmmeter and a volt-meter interposed in the circuits. In observations with 22 patients, measurements have ranged from more than 30 million ohms at the start of a treatment session to 448 ohms with a brain-injured child; voltages have fluctuated between 10 and 254 millivolts. Upledger's interpretation is that the elevation in resistances read with the ohmmeter correlate with the palpable resistances that craniosacral therapists feel with their hands and that the energy put into overcoming these resistances is reflected by elevations in the millivolt readings. On the basis of these preliminary studies, plans are under way to explore further whether the energetic changes measured in the circuits accompany specific landmarks in treatment processes.

References

Upledger, J. E. 1977a. The reproducibility of craniosacral examination findings: a statistical analysis. *J. Am. Osteopath. Assoc.* 76:890–899.

Upledger, J. E. 1977b. The relationship of craniosacral examination findings in grade school children with developmental problems. *J. Am. Osteopath. Assoc.* 77:760–774.

Healing Crisis

DON ASH

One of the best parts of advanced cranial work as taught by The Upledger Institute is that the training requires *you* to do *your own* work. It is with the help of others who are learning and willing to do their own work, that each of us has an opportunity to look at ourselves from different angles offered by the gentle urgings of the CS rhythm. Having said that, it is our decision and ours alone to look, or not to look, at what our bodies are showing us.

I was reminded by a patient today about healing crisis. It refreshed memories of my own healing crisis and essentially the healing that took place because of it.

In my case, I was working as a physical therapist director of rehab services in a small hospital, a part-time home care therapist, a columnist for a local newspaper, a school board member, a volunteer fireman, sheep farmer, husband, and father. To say I was unable to recognize that my life was too hectic was an understatement. So my body tried to help me.

In order for me to see the light, my body gave me a healing crisis. First, I came down with gallbladder disease. So I said, "Okay, take it out and I'll stay home a couple weeks, but then I gotta get back to business." I went back to my schedule and came down with mononucleosis. "Okay," I said, "I'll rest a couple of weeks, but then I gotta get back to work. I've got places to go and people to see."

Reprinted with permission from Don Ash, *Lessons from the Sessions: Reflections of Journeys in CranioSacral Therapy* (Odyssey Press, 22 Nadeau Drive, P.O. Box 7307, Gonic, NH 03839-7307), 77–81.

Then my body became more impatient. I came down with pneumonia and I couldn't breathe. My body was telling me I had to change or go home. No amount of medication or medical intervention in the past twelve months could persuade my body to stop getting my attention. By the way, the pneumonia caused me to cancel a scheduled continuing education course on fascial release work. If someone were to look at my life back in 1987, they would have seen a very successful, committed, highly functioning individual who was taking part in his community and prospering. But the fact is, that life was killing me.

So, I finally realized that I had to alter my life. I was doing too much, moving too fast, and not taking time to balance my life with work, rest, and play. My wonderful body wouldn't stop until I learned this lesson. It needed the length of time it took to break me down. My recovery from pneumonia also coincided with the next available class of fascial release work in my area. The year was 1987, and it was sponsored by an institute I hadn't heard of before. It was The Upledger Institute. So began the process of my healing that forced me to rise out of three health crises to redirect my life. I now know that moving from my very data-based, high stress, institutional setting to having a small CranioSacral practice in an old farm house brought me full circle. Had rapid recovery from my physical problems been achieved with medications, I might not have had the time I needed to process the stress factors in my life, nor discover my passion for the work known as CST.

The lesson from the session here is, it's okay if all of your patients don't have immediate positive response to your treatment. They may be in a healing crisis. Their bodies may need you (the therapist) *to be unsuccessful* in order to allow the patient more time to process the issues of their life. Pain may be a gift from the body encouraging them to change. If we never knew pain, how would we know pleasure? If we never learned bad, how could we recognize good? If we didn't have night, how could we know the absence of darkness is day? How arrogant are we that we think we know what releases need to be released and what emotion needs to be emoted for the greatest good of the patient, and at what time and place this is to occur?

Sometimes the very best we can be, is present. The best we can do, is listen with our hands and facilitate the body to do *what it needs to do* for the patient. It is well to realize that sometimes the best thing we can do for the patient is nothing. Wish them a happy life and move on. In other words, being of no help may be exactly what the patient needs at this time.

As we interact in each other's life, it serves us to realize we can only know that we are somewhere along the patient's path of life. Whether we are on the path or at the crossroads is the great mystery that can only happen when we observe the present moment. Sometimes it is our role to encourage the body to show the person the beginning or the end of their path. It is the young expectant mother's healing crisis that causes her cervix to finally give way and the uterus reach a threshold which begins contractions in an effort to expel the fetus. Sometimes it is the fetus who has a hesitancy to come out of their place of comfort and shelter.

As a PT specializing in CST I occasionally am asked to try CST on an infant considered hopeless. These young souls all have great trouble in landing here on Earth. I consider them great teachers, considering the fact that most of them are less than 6 months old and already they have confounded the greatest medical centers in the world by their very survival.

I held one little man expected to die in the first week of life. He was born with severe anoxia (lack of oxygen to the brain) after a 40 hour home delivery. He required oral suction every 20 minutes. I held him at 9 weeks old. He came to a still point, arched his back, and moaned for

20 minutes. His moan was a heartache and sorrow for his circumstances. He moaned like an old woman that had just lost a son in the war. It came from his solar plexus. His lips puckered, his brow furrowed, his fists clenched, and his little body stiffened. He moaned for his circumstance and then for his right to exist. All of us in the room (mom, other therapist, and myself) felt a chill in our spines as he voiced his healing crisis. He is now one and a half years old, moving all fours. His eyes track. He laughs. He coos. And who's to say he shouldn't live and continue to teach us that life is precious.

Sometimes a healing crisis is the entrance to our exit here on Earth. As it relates to transition, a healing crisis sometimes is the most moving event to allow the notion of death to descend on the person. You know when there is no more life left to live, death (or transition to another existence) is a wonderful alternative to lingering, suffering, and progressive loss of function. When a person is worn down by age or infirmity and fatigued by sleeplessness and exhausted by struggling for breath, there is a gentle curtain that descends and the person quietly resigns. Struggle stops, pain and the grimacing face subside and soften. The mind moves from conflict to acceptance, and vision seems to transcend physical space. Often the person in process sees beyond this physicality and describes the great mystery beyond as bright, warm, and pleasant, with friendly loving faces awaiting.

The healing crisis is the catalyst for awareness shift, in that the stimulation doesn't quit, until the patient does, and then there is calm, peace, and transition.

And from personal, first-hand witness experience, I can tell you, after the last breath, and the heart stops, the last physically perceivable movement in the entire body is the cranial rhythm that trails off to a whisper and is gone.

The Chinese express crisis with two symbols, one for danger and one for opportunity. Another lesson from the session here is: We are charged as CST therapists to stand with the patient in the perceived moment of risk and watch for the opportunity to understand and experience this life. Ours is not to know if they are coming or going, only that it is sacred.

Self-Discovery and Self-Healing

JOHN E. UPLEDGER

The secret something that is shared by all effective healing methods can perhaps be best characterized as the process of leading the patient to an honest and truthful self-discovery. This self-discovery is required for the initiation and continuation of self-healing; for it is only through self-healing—in contrast to "curing"—that patients can experience both permanent recovery and spiritual growth.

Before discussing self-discovery and self-healing, however, we need to examine the meanings of the terms *healing* and *curing*. The distinction between the two defines a developing polarity in the thinking of health-care professionals. The two words share essentially the same definition in dictionaries, both referring to a method or course of remedial treatment that aims to restore health. Yet this official definition does not capture the implications that the two words have taken in today's health-care world.

At present we often use the term *healing* to refer to what is done *by* the patient (or the patient's body) in order to resolve a problem of the body, mind, or spirit; whereas the term *curing* usually refers to what is done *to* the patient by a physician or therapist. So we frequently speak of patients as needing to "heal themselves" after the disease has been "cured." Surgical removal of the gallbladder, for instance, may

Reprinted with permission from Richard Carlson and Benjamin Shield, eds., *Healers on Healing* (New York: Jeremy P. Tarcher, 1989), 67–72.

"cure" gallbladder disease, but the patient must then "heal" the wound and adapt to the absence of that organ in order to achieve adequate function of the digestive system.

The reason we need to clarify the difference between healing and curing is quite simple: Effective therapy—whatever its outer form— initiates, facilitates, and supports the patient's self-healing efforts, whereas the "curing" process is one that provides a more temporary and perhaps only palliative effect. Although "curing" may remove the symptoms of a disease from the outside, so to speak, it usually leaves the underlying causes of the symptoms untouched.

For example, a physician might "cure" hemorrhoids by surgically removing them. If, however, the hemorrhoids are secondary to a congested liver that is due to chronic drinking, the problem will not be "healed" until the patient resolves the underlying reason for the alcohol abuse. In this case, it might be better for the surgeon to leave the hemorrhoids intact, as a reminder and perhaps motivating force that will help focus the patient's attention on the alcohol abuse. In this way the real cause of the problem may one day be eradicated.

A friend and general surgeon with more than thirty years' experience once confided to me that, in retrospect, he felt the majority of surgical procedures he had performed might be classified as excisions of the "vocal apparatuses" of the inner selves of his patients. He meant that by removing certain organs or tissues, he was eliminating the bodily voices that were attempting to communicate the presence of deeper emotional or spiritual problems in need of attention.

Thus, to refer again to our previous example of an alcohol-abusing hemorrhoid patient, we must consider that although removal of the hemorrhoids might temporarily alleviate some of the symptoms, it also removes one avenue by which the inner self is attempting to focus attention on the alcohol problem. If the hemorrhoids are removed and the alcohol abuse continues, the inner self has no choice but to select another organ to use as an attention-getter.

The next "target" organ might be the gallbladder. The next step will be for the surgeon to remove the gallbladder, which may be full of gallstones. Certainly the surgeon feels justified in performing both surgeries, yet no attempt has been made to determine whether the patient's inner self is trying to relay some underlying message to the conscious mind. So we now have a heavily drinking patient without hemorrhoids or gallbladder who still has little or no idea why he or she is abusing alcohol. Perhaps the drinking is a means of escape from guilt feelings instilled during childhood by a parent. If so, the issue is left unexplored and the abuse continues until, eventually, the function of the liver begins to falter.

As the deterioration proceeds, the "inner voice" of the body's wisdom will feel an increasingly urgent need to contact the patient's conscious mind. So it is likely that varicose veins will develop in the esophagus. The situation is now serious and life-threatening, requiring co-management by internal medicine specialists as well as surgeons. Once these veins are surgically dealt with, there is little remaining that can be removed, except the liver itself in the rare cases when a transplant may be undertaken. Usually, however, the internist must support the abused and failing liver until death intervenes.

Let's backtrack a little. Somewhere along the line, a psychiatrist may have been called in to deal with the compulsive alcohol abuse, or because the patient may have been recognized as suicidal. In either case, most of the drugs prescribed by the psychiatrist will probably have both mind-altering and hepatotoxic (liver-poisoning) qualities. Therefore, the "inner voice" will have even less chance of communicating with the drug-compromised conscious mind about the reason for the alcohol abuse (i.e., unresolved guilt), and the liver function will be further impaired by the toxic nature of the drugs. Finally, premature death occurs.

The cause of death will probably be recorded as "liver failure due to alcohol abuse." From our perspective, however, it might be as accurate to say that the cause of death was the hemorrhoidectomy performed without search for an underlying message or cause; or the second excision of the "inner voice," which was attempting to speak through the gallbladder.

Becoming aware of this inner voice is what I mean by the kind of self-discovery that leads to self-healing. In the case just discussed, treatment not only failed to make the patient aware of the inner voice, it ultimately suppressed it. This treatment led to a self-perpetuating cycle of deterioration. Short of a miracle, the process was probably not reversible once the varicose veins developed in the esophagus and the brain was numbed by mind-altering drugs. After all, what chance does the inner voice have against modern surgical technology and psychopharmacology?

In response to the failure of traditional "curing" methods to provide meaningful assistance to those struggling with deeper problems that manifest as body dysfunctions, a myriad of health-related treatment techniques, methods, and philosophies have been created. These include a wide spectrum of practices, such as meditation, nutritional therapy, herbal therapy, homeopathy, acupuncture, Rolfing, chiropractic, Alexander-Feldenkrais technique, rebirthing, counseling, biofeedback, to name a few. Each of these systems, although outwardly different, facilitates the self-discovery that leads to self-healing.

In considering how the process of self-discovery works, it is important to remember that our self-image is constantly changing. It seems that the closer our perception of self approaches the truth, the deeper our capacity for self-healing becomes. When there is a very close correspondence between self-image and truth, our self-healing power may be virtually unlimited, capable of producing the "miracle cure." So, the main responsibility of the therapist is to help the patient develop a truer, more correct self-image.

This means that when working with a patient, the therapist must become an accurate reflecting mirror, a medium through which the patient's real self can be perceived more clearly. This true self-image may not be compatible with the therapist's preconceived notion of the patient's problem, if such a preconceived notion exists. The therapist must become an unbiased facilitator. Then the truth can be discovered by both patient and therapist.

In order to allow for this discovery, the facilitator must remove, as much as possible, the influences of ego and any tendency to engage in diagnostic cataloging. The facilitator can then become a clear reflecting medium that permits no illusion, delusion, camouflage, or facade.

During this process, the facilitator cannot force too much perception of truth at one time or the patient may turn away from the reflection. Therefore, the "mirror" must be very sensitive, reflecting only as much as the patient is able to deal with at any given time. Still, it must reflect enough to prevent stagnation and keep the self-discovery process moving. The art of therapy is in sensing how rapidly the process can move without creating resistance or turning the patient away, and in allowing the patient to make his or her own discoveries. This art requires that the therapist avoid suggestion and leading. It also involves a connection with the patient at an unconscious level. The process of self-discovery may continue with or without words.

My own therapeutic style uses physical touch to facilitate the establishment of a connection between myself and the patient's unconscious. Other therapists may establish this connection by other means, but for me it is the act of touching, of physical contact between myself and the patient, that allows me to establish this communication.

As I blend or merge with the patient by the use of touch, I make every effort to remain open to any perceptions, sensations, or insights that may penetrate into my conscious awareness from the patient. I believe that every organ, tissue, and cell in the body has its own consciousness. This is usually not within the scope of the patient's conscious awareness. However, when I remain open, I receive information from these unconscious parts. These messages may enter my conscious mind as pain in my own body, a visual image, a verbal message, or a sort of knowing or insight that circumvents contributing clues and information fragments along the way.

For example, our patient with the liver problem from alcohol abuse may cause me to experience discomfort in my own liver; or I may see a visual image of a damaged liver; or I may hear the patient's unconscious voice telling me that his liver is damaged; or I may sense that he is a problem drinker due to parent-instilled guilt. When this information is received, my goal is to assist the patient in self-discovery so that he knows that the symptoms are due to alcohol abuse, and why the alcohol abuse came about and why it continues.

The process of communication between patient and therapist is stimulated by the act of touching with intent to assist in the healing process. This patient-therapist communication is initially on an unconscious level. Then it usually emerges into the therapist's conscious awareness. The therapist then works to assist the patient in developing an awareness of the information received. For it is when the patient is consciously informed that he or she can best do something intelligent about the problem. Therefore, in my own practice, I try very hard to reflect a true picture, to be an honest yet sensitive mirror. The patient does not have to see the truth all at once, but I do not aid and abet the continuance of an illusion, unless (as happens in rare cases) it seems very important for the patient to maintain this illusion—and then only for the time necessary for adaption and growth to occur.

When the process of self-discovery has resulted in genuine self-healing, it may or may not produce a "cure"—that is, the elimination of symptoms. For true healing goes deeper than symptoms; it involves getting clear about your real identity and purpose in life. For this reason, healing may sometimes mean spending the rest of your life in a wheelchair—if that is how you can best perform your life task. You may be "healed" even though you remain in a wheelchair, providing you recognize that this is how things are supposed to be for you. Similarly, healing may mean recognizing that it is okay to die. It may mean that the problems and conflicts posed to you for solution during this lifetime have been resolved and that you are now free to leave this environment.

So the successful therapeutic process does not necessarily produce comfort, ease, muscular strength, prolonged life, or any of the other things that our Western medical tradition has come to hold as evidence of healing. Effective therapy does, however, give the individual patient a clear vision of what he or she needs to do, as well as the strength and integration of mind, body, and spirit to do it. The goals of therapy are the elimination of delusion and self-pity and the helping of patients to prioritize and focus their lives so that they can grow.

In the therapeutic process the single most important factor seems to be the ability of the therapist to reflect back the truth to the patient. For it is truth that heals. Truth is the golden thread found in all effective therapeutic systems.

Glossary

Allopathy. A method of treating disease with remedies that produce effects different from those caused by the disease itself. This was the term applied by homeopaths to traditional medicine.

Arcing. A technique that requires the practitioner to sense the energetic waves of interference produced by an active lesion/problem. Practitioners then trace these waves to their source by manually sensing the arcs that they form.

Bioenergetics. A school of therapy that seeks to relieve stress and concomitant muscular tension through respiratory exercises, physical movement, improvement in body image, and free expression of ideas.

Cerebral palsy. A persisting qualitative motor dysfunction that appears before the age of three years. It is due to non-progressive damage to the brain, which in turn could be due to any one of a number of causes.

Cerebrospinal fluid. The plasma-like fluid that is extracted from blood by the choroids plexus within the brain's ventricular system. It is contained within the compartment formed by the dura mater. The functions of cerebrospinal fluid still offer several mysteries to modern science. We know that it offers a hydraulic cushion for the brain to soften the blows of the delicate brain and spinal cord against their bony containers during accidents and so on. Also, the cerebrospinal fluid supplies some nutrition, removes some waste, and perhaps provides some acid-alkaline balance stability for the brain and spinal cord. There is also some conjecture that it contains an inherent energy.

Coccyx. Triangular bone formed by fusion of the last four (sometimes three or five) vertebrae at the extreme lower end of the spinal column during fetal development.

Cranial osteopathy. Developed by William Garner Sutherland, this technique involves a gentle manipulation of the skull to relieve tension and pain, bringing the body back into harmony.

Cranium. The skull, made up of twenty-one bones. The bones are the occiput, two parietal bones, two temporal bones, frontal, sphenoid, two maxilla, mandible, two zygoma, two palatines, one vomer, one ethmoid, two lacrimals, two nasal bones, and the inferior nasal concha.

Cytoskeleton. The inner structural elements, or backbone, of a cell. It consists of microtubules and various filaments that spread out through the cytoplasm, providing both structural support and a means of transport within the cell.

Dura mater. Also known as the dural membrane, it is the outermost, toughest of three meninges (membranes) which form the sac or envelope which contains the brain and the spinal cord.

Dural membrane. Also known as the dura mater, it is the outermost, toughest of three meninges (membranes) which form the sac or envelope which contains the brain and the spinal cord.

Embryology. The branch of biology that deals with the formation, early growth, and development of living organisms.

Energy Cyst. The imprint of physical or emotional trauma that is retained in the body and transmits its restrictive effects fascially throughout the body.

Entropy. The negative energy that causes things to age, ultimately die, or fall apart.

Fascia. A thin layer of connective tissue covering, supporting, and connecting various structures of the body; one continuous sheet throughout the body.

Homeopathy. A nontraditional system for treating and preventing disease, in which minute amounts of a substance that in large amounts causes disease symptoms are given to healthy individuals. This is thought to enhance the body's natural defenses.

Lamina. A thin layer of bone, membrane, or other tissue.

Lesion. A region of local damage to the nervous system. Lesions occur as a result of diseases, such as strokes, which destroy nerve cell bodies and axons.

Meninges. The three membranes covering the brain and spinal cord: dura mater, arachnoid membrane, and pia mater.

Motility. The capacity of or exhibition of spontaneous motion and breathing of the fluids of the body of the Tide and the soma, including each bone and organ.

Myofascial. Of or relating to the fascia surrounding and separating muscle tissue.

Myofascial Release. A form of bodywork which includes, but is not limited to structural assessments and manual massage techniques for stretching the fascia and releasing bonds between fascia. The goal of this technique is to eliminate pain, increase range of motion, and restore balance to the body.

Occiput. The back part of the head. Also used to denote the occipital bone, which forms the posterior part of the skull vault and part of the floor of the skull cavity.

Osteopathy. Originally founded by Andrew Taylor Still, this system of primary care is based on the theory that the body is capable of healing itself. It emphasizes a holistic approach and the skilled use of a range of manual and physical treatment interventions.

Palpate. Examine by touch; that which can be touched or felt.

Parietal bone. One of a pair of bones forming the top and sides of the cranium.

Poise. The resting attitude of the organism.

Polarity. A therapy developed by Dr. Randolph Stone that uses touch, verbal interaction, exercise, nutrition, and other methods. A primary focus is on re-establishing balance in the central nervous system.

Reflexive sympathetic dystrophy (RSD). A painful condition that results from the sympathetic nervous system going out of control.

Sacrum. A curved triangular bone located at the base of the lumbar spine, consisting of five fused vertebra; dural tube ends at the second sacral segment.

SomatoEmotional Release (SER). The release of suppressed emotion that has resulted from a physical or emotional trauma.

Sutures. A stitch or series of stitches made to secure apposition of the edges of a surgical or traumatic wound. Also, the joint between two skull bones. Skull sutures are slightly moveable throughout life except under pathological conditions. Sutural mobility is one of the corner stones of craniosacral therapy.

Temporomandibular joint syndrome (TMJ). A painful problem caused by the joints of the lower jaw becoming dysfunctional. Some possible causes include an imbalance between the temporal bones on each side of the head, nervous tension that results in tooth grinding and/or jaw clenching, whiplash injury to the neck, or a malocclusion of the teeth.

Thorax. The part of the human body between the neck and the diaphragm, partially encased by the ribs and containing the heart and lungs; the chest.

Tide. Traditional term used synonymously with Long Tide, Primary Respiration, and Primary Respiratory Impulse. It was originally coined by William Garner Sutherland to describe the rhythmic ebb and flow of the cerebrospinal fluid and the potency in the flow.

Trauma. A physiological or psychic response to physical, emotional, or spiritual injury. It is usually the result of being overwhelmed by shock and not having resources available to integrate the shock; thus trauma occurs and becomes embedded in the mind-body continuum.

Viscera. The soft internal organs of the body, especially those contained within the abdominal and thoracic cavities.

Visceral Manipulation. A type of osteopathic manipulative therapy that involves making contact with the internal organs, especially those in the abdomen, in an attempt to relieve somatic dysfunction.

Zero Balancing. A hands-on bodywork system designed to align the energy body with the physical structure. It incorporates Eastern concepts of energy and healing.

About the Authors

John E. Upledger, DO, OMM, is president and founder of The Upledger Institute, Inc. Dedicated to the natural enhancement of health, the Institute is recognized worldwide for its groundbreaking continuing-education programs, clinical research, and therapeutic services.

Throughout his career as an osteopathic physician, Dr. Upledger has been recognized as an innovator and leading proponent in the investigation of new therapies. His development of CranioSacral Therapy in particular has earned him an international reputation. TIME magazine named him one of the world's next wave of innovators in 2001. He has also served on the Alternative Medicine Program Advisory Council for the Office of Alternative Medicine at the National Institutes of Health in Washington, D.C.

Dr. Upledger is a Certified Specialist of Osteopathic Manipulative Medicine, an Academic Fellow of the British Society of Osteopathy, and a Doctor of Science in alternative medicine. He has written numerous textbooks and study guides, more than two dozen research articles, and he is a regular contributor and columnist for national publications dedicated to manual therapy.

Richard Grossinger is a graduate of Amherst College and has a PhD in anthropology from the University of Michigan. He is the author of numerous books, including *Planet Medicine* and *Embryogenesis: Species, Gender, and Identity.* He studied craniosacral therapy with Randy Cherner and through The Upledger Institute during the early 1990s.

Don Ash has been a physical therapist for over thirty years. He now specializes in craniosacral therapy and has a small practice in rural seacoast New Hampshire. He is the author of *Lessons from the Sessions: Reflections of Journeys in CranioSacral Therapy*. Most recently, he contributed a section on craniosacral therapy for *New Foundations in Therapeutic Massage and Bodywork*. He has also contributed to several books by Dr. Upledger and he teaches nationally and internationally for The Upledger Institute.

Don Cohen, DC, is a graduate of Palmer College of Chiropractic West and of The Upledger Institute. Since 1982 he has practiced chiropractic and craniosacral therapy in Santa Cruz, California, with his wife Karen, a constitutional homeopath. Since 1985 he has been engaged in clinical research into the relationship of neurologic adaptation strategy to musculoskeletal injury, chronic pain, and degeneration syndromes. He is working on a forthcoming book, *Neural Logic: The Strategies of Adaptation*.

About North Atlantic Books

North Atlantic Books (NAB) is an independent, nonprofit publisher committed to a bold exploration of the relationships between mind, body, spirit, and nature. Founded in 1974, NAB aims to nurture a holistic view of the arts, sciences, humanities, and healing. To make a donation or to learn more about our books, authors, events, and newsletter, please visit www.northatlanticbooks.com.

North Atlantic Books is the publishing arm of the Society for the Study of Native Arts and Sciences, a 501(c)(3) nonprofit educational organization that promotes cross-cultural perspectives linking scientific, social, and artistic fields. To learn how you can support us, please visit our website.